WORKBOOK

ILLUSTRATED

Dental Embryology, Histology, AND Anatomy

SECOND EDITION

MARY BATH-BALOGH, BA, BS, MS

Faculty, Department Coordinator
Department of Biological Sciences
Pierce College, Lakewood, Washington

MARGARET J. FEHRENBACH, RDH, MS

Oral Biologist and Dental Hygienist
Adjunct Faculty Position, Marquette University, Milwaukee, Wisconsin
Educational Consultant and Private Practice, Seattle, Washington

Illustrated by

PAT THOMAS, CMI

Certified Medical Illustrator, AMI
Oak Park, Illinois

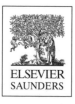

ELSEVIER
SAUNDERS

ELSEVIER
SAUNDERS

11830 Westline Industrial Drive
St. Louis, Missouri 63146

ISBN-13: 978-1-4160-3471-1
ISBN-10: 1-4160-3471-4

Publishing Director: Linda Duncan
Executive Editor: Penny Rudolph
Developmental Editor: Courtney Sprehe
Publishing Services Manager: Melissa Lastarria
Project Manager: Ellen Kunkelmann
Designer: Teresa McBryan

Printed in the United States of America

Last digit is the print number: 9 8 7 6 5 4

PREFACE

This companion to *Illustrated Dental Embryology, Histology, and Anatomy* provides a wide range of activities and skill-building exercises to strengthen student readers' understanding of the principles discussed in the main text. It includes graph paper templates and evaluation criteria to help when drawing teeth. It also has structure identification exercises, glossary exercises, case studies, information on infection control and occlusal evaluation, and removable tooth identification flashcards.

Additional study material can also found online on the associated Evolve website. The website features chapter discussion questions, supplemental study materials, an update section that explores developments in the field, and web links to increase interest in the subject. We hope that this material will help students be able to more easily integrate their knowledge into clinical dental coursework.

Mary Bath-Balogh
Margaret J. Fehrenbach

TABLE OF CONTENTS

Structure

Identification

Exercises

Unit I:
Introduction to
Dental Structures

Chapter 1: Face and Neck Regions

Directions: When examining a peer, check off the items noted in an extraoral examination of both sides of a normal face and neck. Use both visual inspection and palpation. Include the lymph nodes of the face and neck also, if applicable.

Regions of the Face	
Frontal, Orbital and Nasal Regions	
Forehead	
Orbits	
External Nose: Root of Nose, Apex of Nose, Nares, Nasal Septum, Nasal Alae	
Infraorbital and Zygomatic Regions	
Zygomatic Arches	
Temporomandibular Joints	
Buccal Regions	
Cheeks and Masseter Muscles	
Angles of the Mandible	
Parotid Salivary Glands	
Oral Region	
Lips: Vermilion Zones and Borders	
Philtrum	
Tubercle of Upper Lip	
Labial Commissures	
Nasolabial Sulcus (on each side)	
Labiomental Groove	

Structure Identification Exercise for Chapter 1: Face and Neck Regions (*continued*):

Mental Region and Lower Face	
Mandible (on each side): Ramus, Coronoid Process, Coronoid Notch, Condyle, Mandibular Notch	
Regions of the Neck	
Sternocleidomastoid muscles	
Hyoid Bone	
Thyroid Cartilage	
Thyroid Gland	
Submandibular Salivary Glands	
Sublingual Salivary Glands	

Chapter 2: Oral Cavity and Pharynx

Directions: When examining a peer, check off the items noted in an intraoral examination of both sides of a normal oral cavity and pharynx. Use both visual inspection and palpation. Also note normal variations such as Fordyce's spots, linea alba, exostoses, mandibular tori, and palatal torus, if applicable. The base of the tongue and its structures, such as the lingual tonsil, are usually not visible when examining the oral cavity. Note also the relationship of the nasopharynx and laryngopharynx to the oropharynx, even though they are also not visible.

Oral Cavity	
Vestibules	
Labial Mucosa	
Buccal Mucosa and Buccal Fat Pads	
Parotid Papillae	
Parotid Salivary Glands	
Vestibular Fornix	
Alveolar Mucosa	
Labial Frenum: Maxillary and Mandibular	
Jaws, Alveolar Processes, Teeth and Dental Arches	
Maxilla: Maxillary Sinuses, Alveolar Process, Alveoli, Canine Eminences, Maxillary Teeth, Maxillary Tuberosities	
Mandible: Alveolar Process, Alveoli, Canine Eminences, Mandibular Teeth, Retromolar Pads	
Teeth: Crown, Enamel (Note other portions in relationship to these portions), Incisors, Canines, Premolars, and Molars	

Structure Identification Exercise for Chapter 2: Oral Cavity and Pharynx (*continued*):

Gingiva and Associated Structures	
Attached Gingiva	
Mucogingival Junction	
Marginal Gingiva	
Gingival Sulcus (location only)	
Interdental Gingiva	
Oral Cavity Proper	
Fauces	
Anterior Faucial Pillars	
Posterior Faucial Pillars	
Palatine Tonsils	
Palate	
Hard Palate	
Median Palatine Raphe	
Incisive Papilla	
Palatine Rugae	
Uvula of the Palate	
Soft Palate	
Pterygomandibular Folds	
Tongue	
Base of Tongue (anterior portion only)	
Body of Tongue	
Dorsal Surface	
Median Lingual Sulcus	
Filiform Lingual Papillae	
Fungiform Lingual Papillae	
Sulcus Terminalis and Foramen Cecum (if possible)	
Circumvallate Lingual Papillae	
Lateral Surfaces	
Foliate Lingual Papillae	
Ventral Surface	
Plica Fimbriatae	

Structure Identification Exercise for Chapter 2: Oral Cavity and Pharynx (*continued*):

Floor of the Mouth	
Lingual Frenum	
Sublingual Folds	
Sublingual Salivary Glands	
Submandibular Salivary Glands	
Sublingual Caruncles	
Pharynx	
Oropharynx	

Unit II: Dental Embryology

Chapter 3: Overview of Prenatal Development

1. Figure 3-4

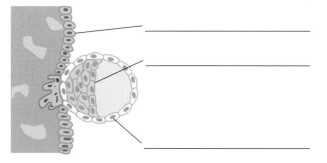

2. Figure 3-6

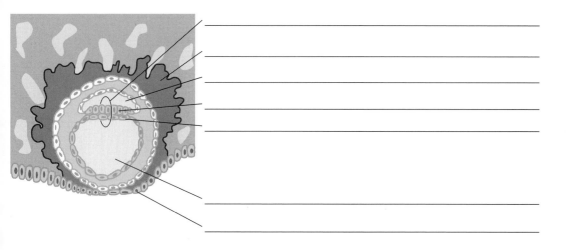

3. Figure 3-7

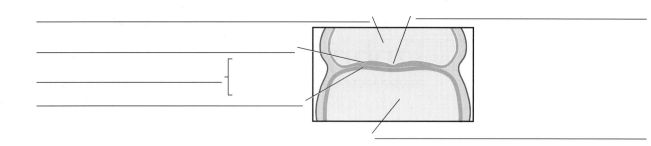

4. Figure 3-8

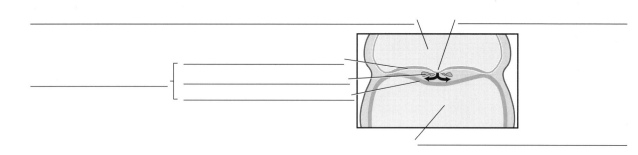

5. Figure 3-9

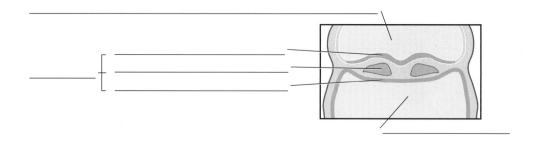

6. Figure 3-10 A

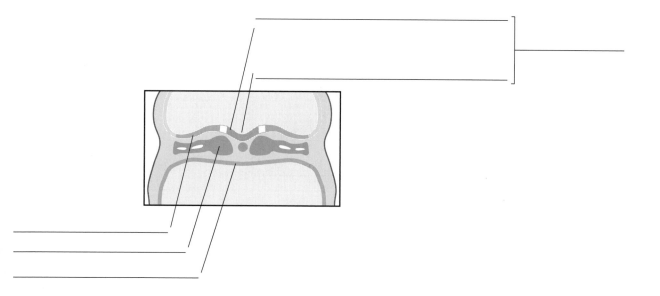

7. Figure 3-10 B

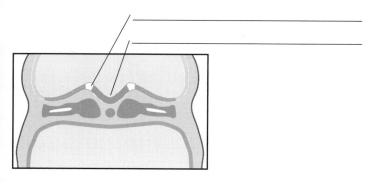

8. Figure 3-10 C

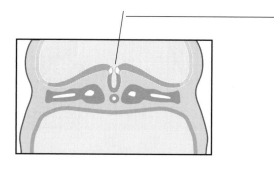

9.   Figure 3-11 A

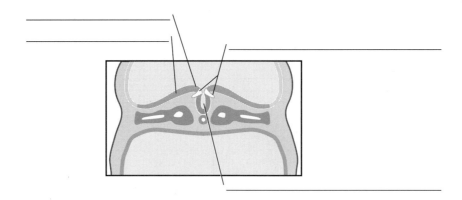

10.   Figure 3-11 B

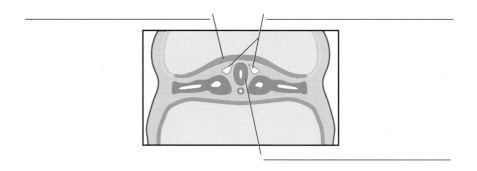

11.   Figure 3-14

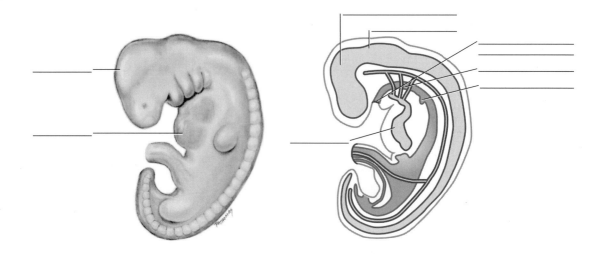

Chapter 4: Development of the Face and Neck

12.   Figure 4-1

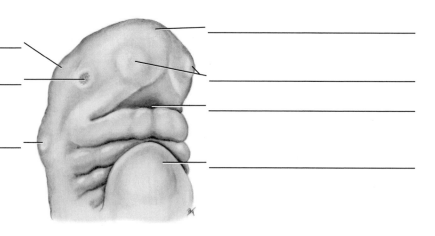

_____

_____

_____

13.   Figure 4-3

Embryonic Derivatives

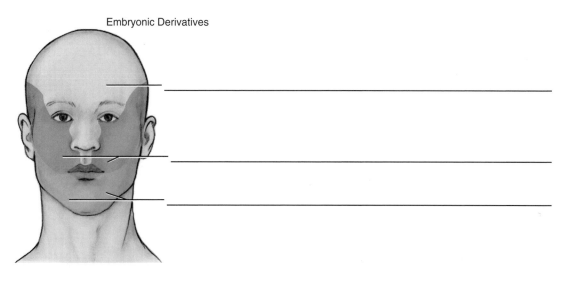

14. Figure 4-5

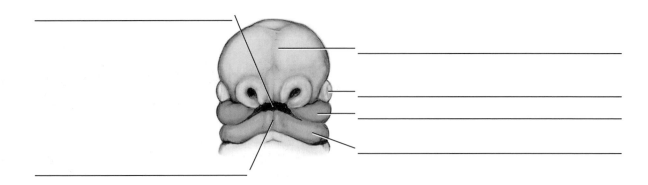

15. Figure 4-6

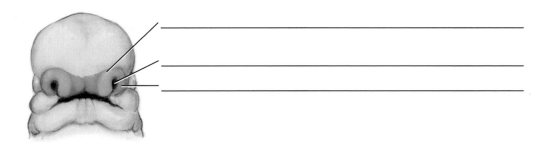

Chapter 5: Development of Orofacial Structures

16.   Figure 5-2

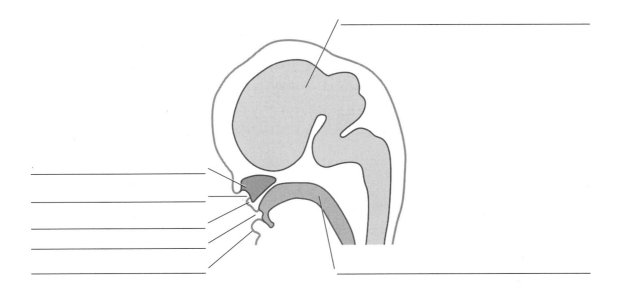

17.   Figure 5-3

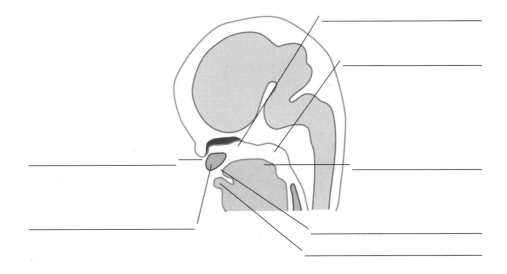

18. Figure 5-4 A

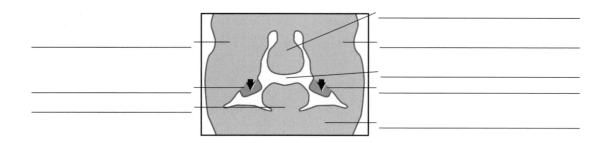

19. Figure 5-4 C

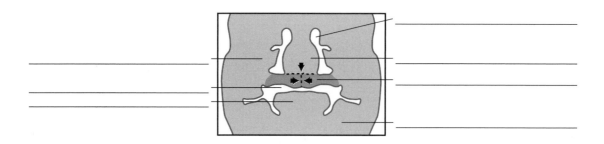

20. Figure 5-6

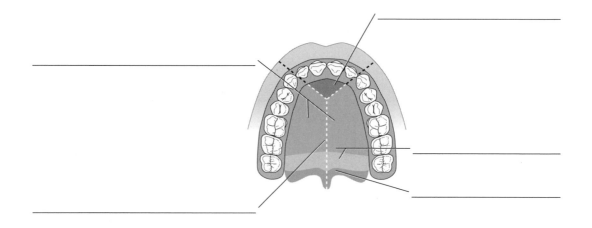

21. Figure 5-10 A

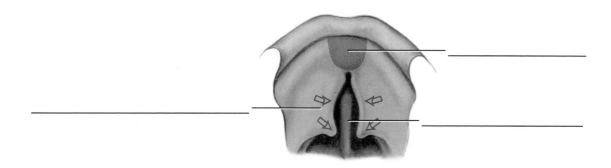

22. Figure 5-10 B

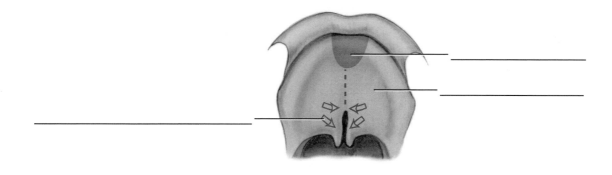

23. Figure 5-10 C

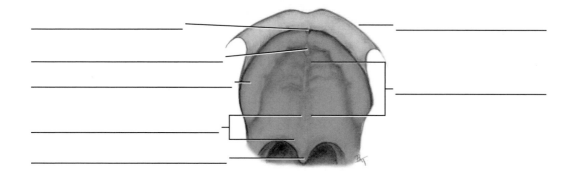

Chapter 6: Tooth Development and Eruption

24.   Figure 6-2

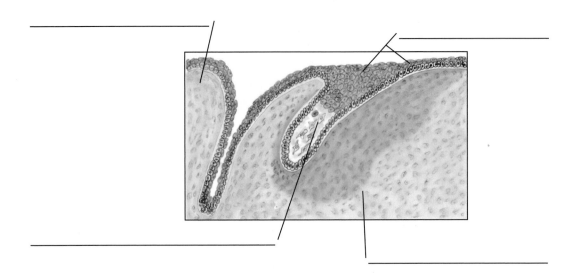

25.   Figure 6-3

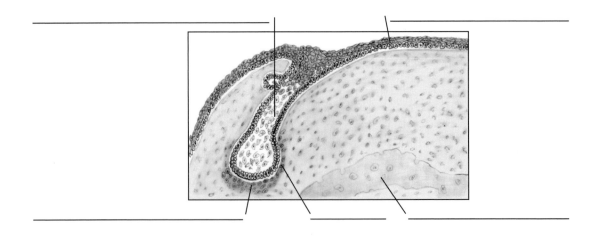

26.   Figure 6-5

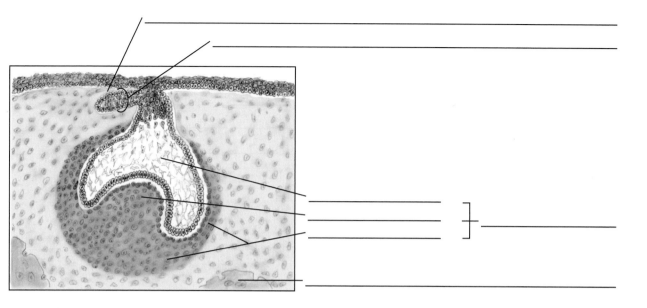

27.   Figure 6-7

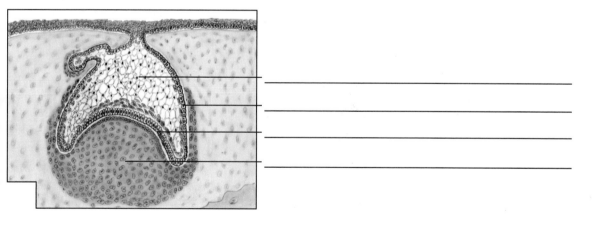

28.　Figure 6-7

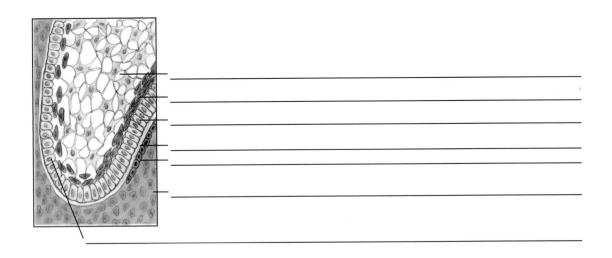

29.　Figure 6-12

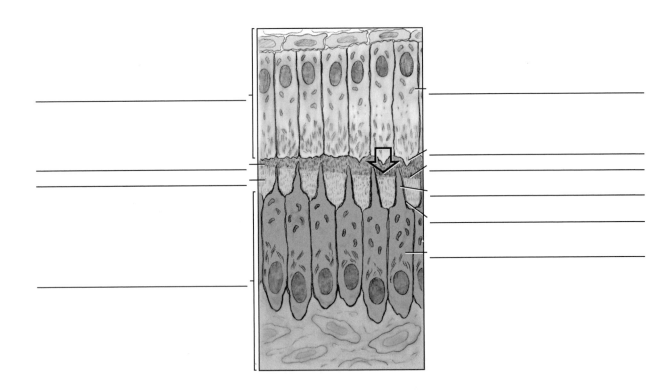

30. Figure 6-13

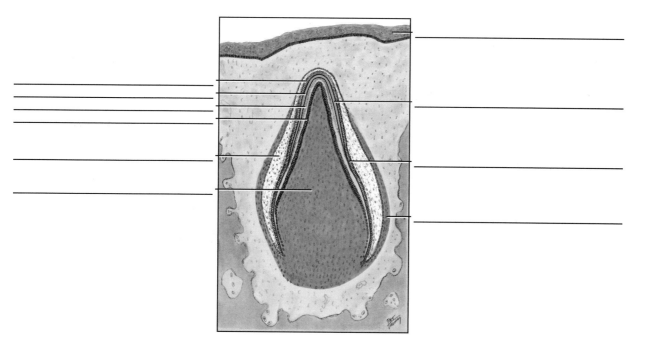

31. Figure 6-18 A

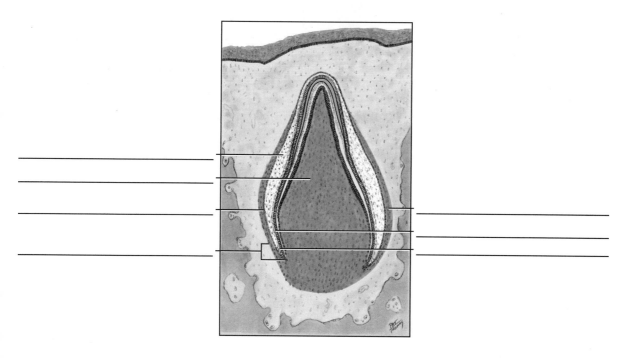

32. Figure 6-18 B

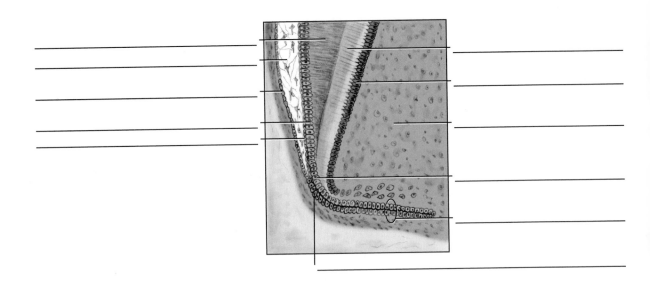

33. Figure 6-19

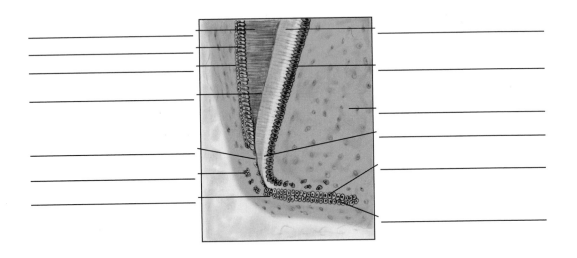

34.   Figure 6-20

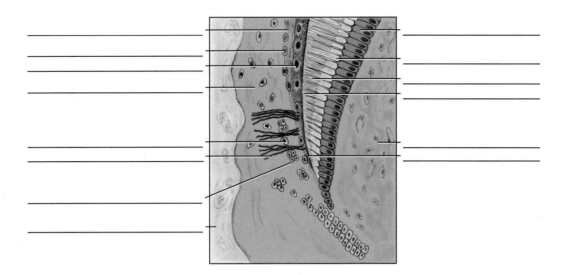

35.   Figure 6-27

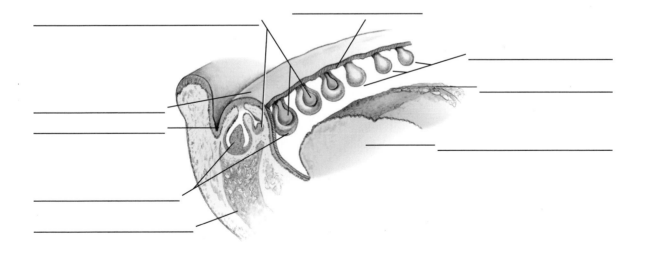

Unit III: Dental Histology

Chapter 7: Overview of the Cell

1. Figure 7-2

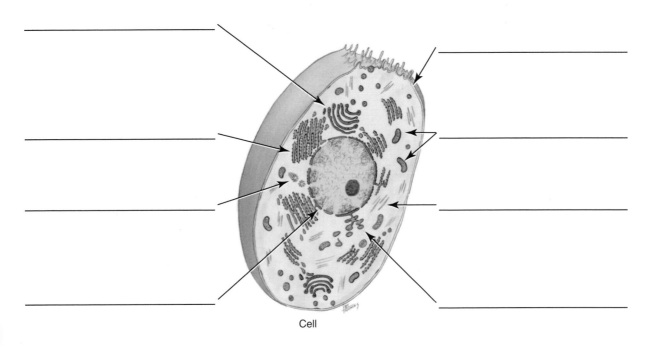

Cell

2. Figure 7-3

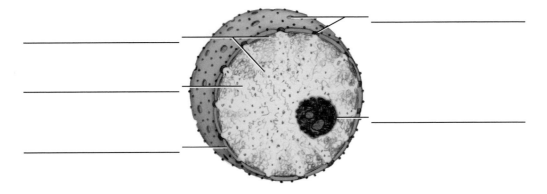

Chapter 8: Basic Tissues

3. Figure 8-4

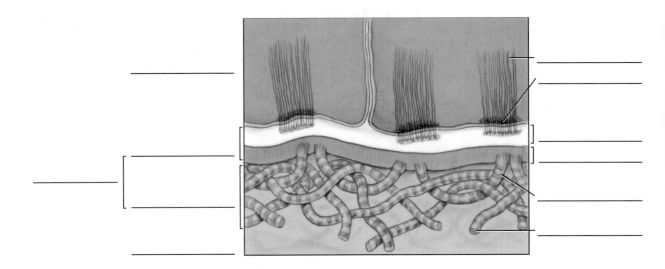

4. Figure 8-7

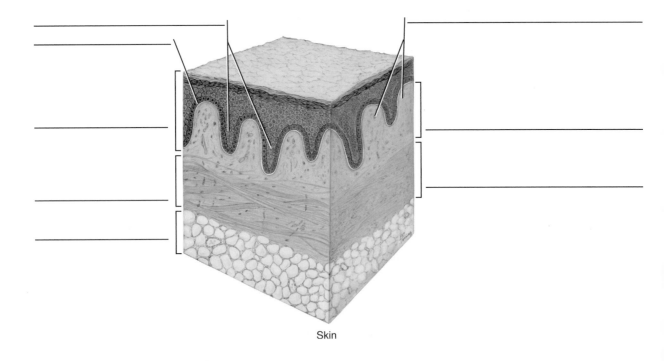

Skin

5.   Figure 8-8

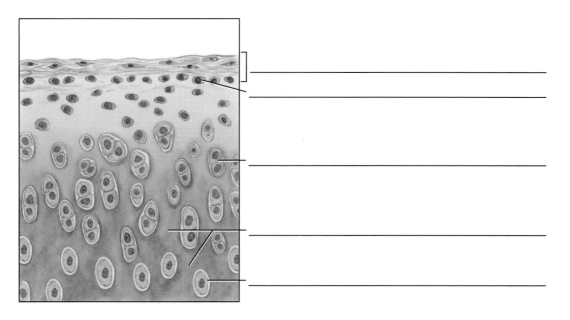

6.   Figure 8-9

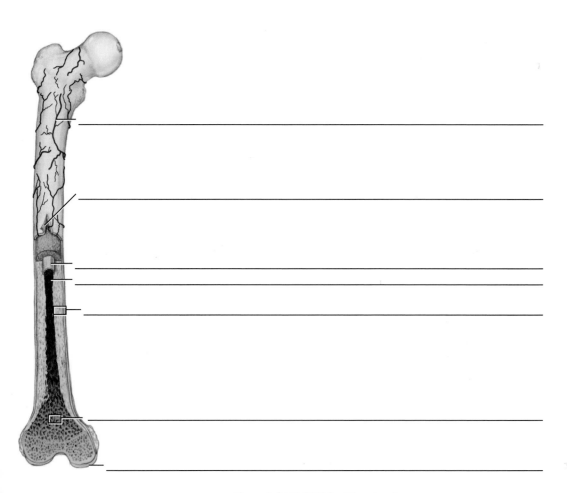

7. Figure 8-10

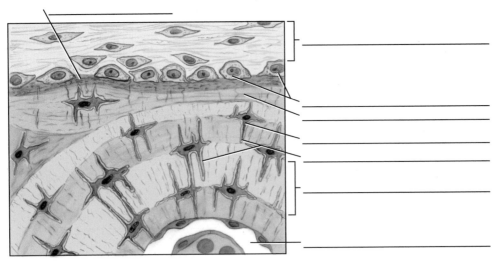

Diagram of the Histology of Bone

8. Figure 8-15

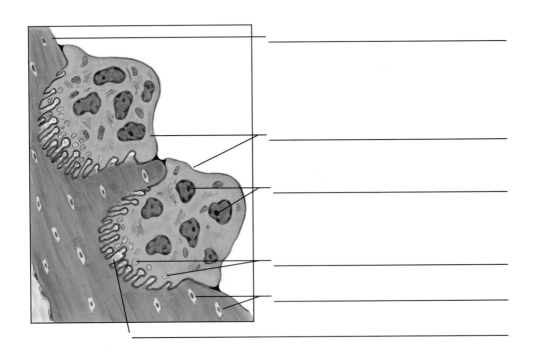

Chapter 9: Oral Mucosa

9. Figure 9-1

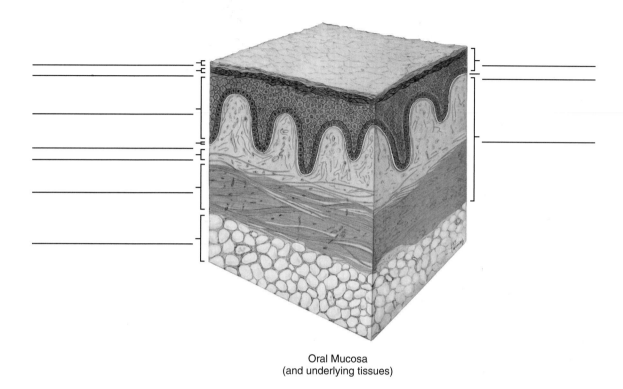

Oral Mucosa
(and underlying tissues)

10. Figure 9-2

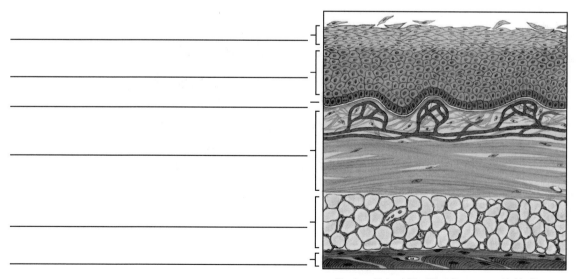

Nonkeratinized Stratified Squamous Epithelium
(and deeper tissues)

11. Figure 9-3

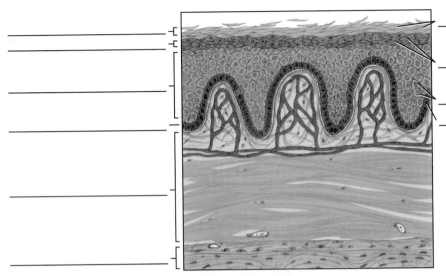

Orthokeratinized Stratified Squamous Epithelium
(and deeper tissues)

12. Figure 9-5

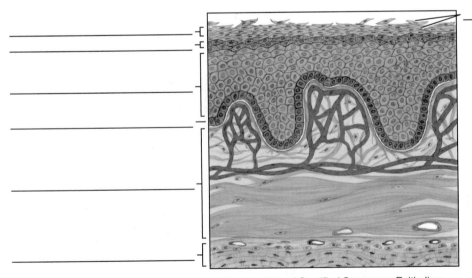

Parakeratinized Stratified Squamous Epithelium
(and deeper tissues)

13. Figure 9-7

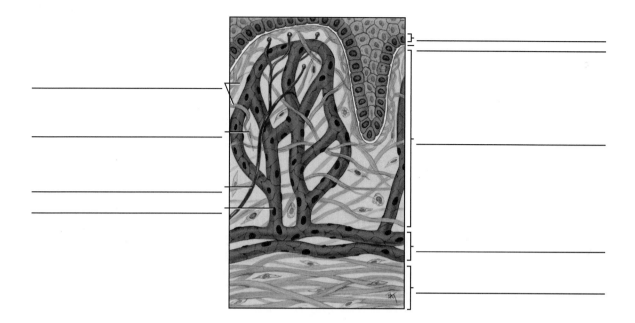

14. Figure 9-16

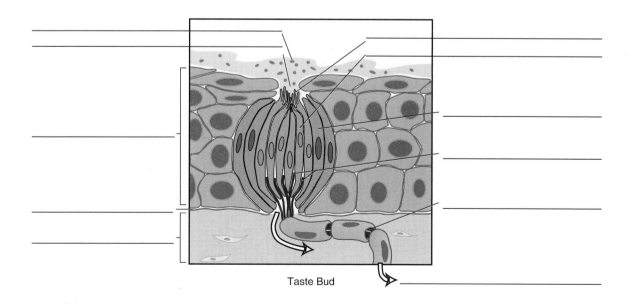

Taste Bud

Chapter 10: Gingival and Dentogingival Junctional Tissues

15. Figure 10-1

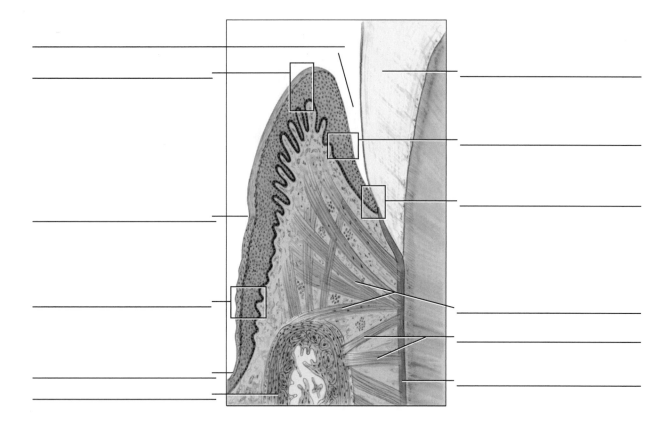

16. Figure 10-8

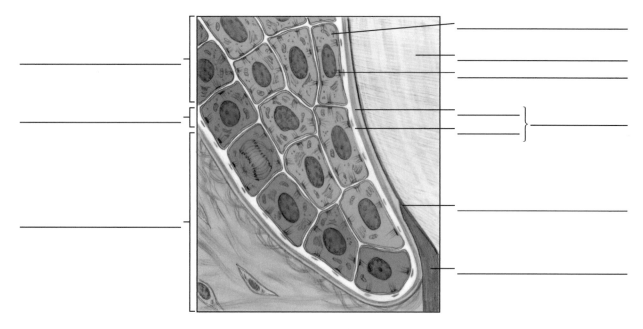

Chapter 11: Head and Neck Structures

17. Figure 11-1

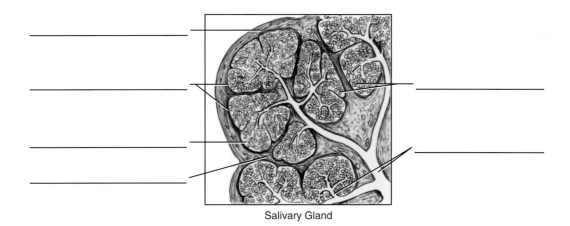

Salivary Gland

18. Figure 11-6

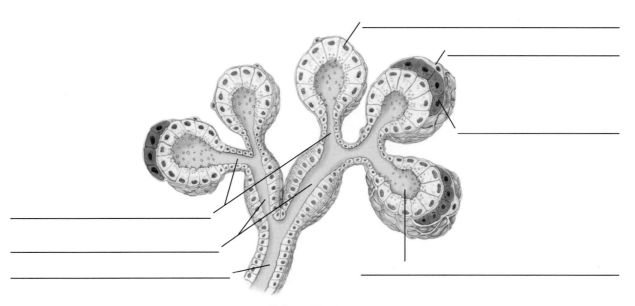

Salivary Gland

19. Figure 11-13

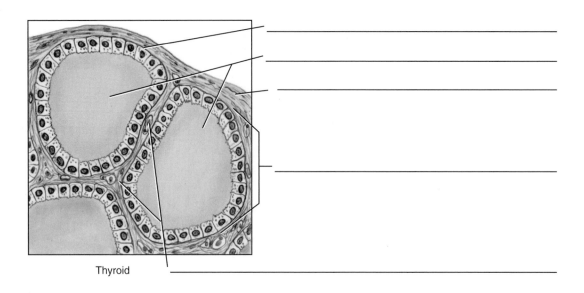

Thyroid

20. Figure 11-16

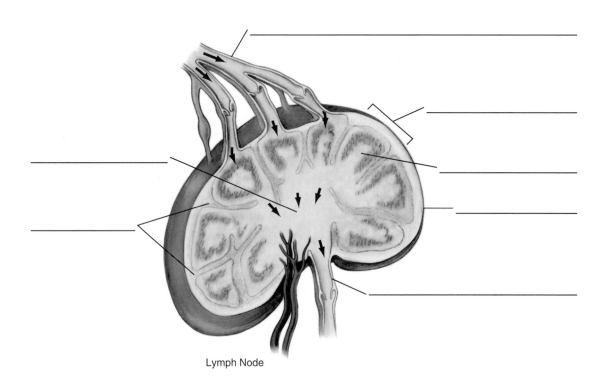

Lymph Node

21. Figure 11-17

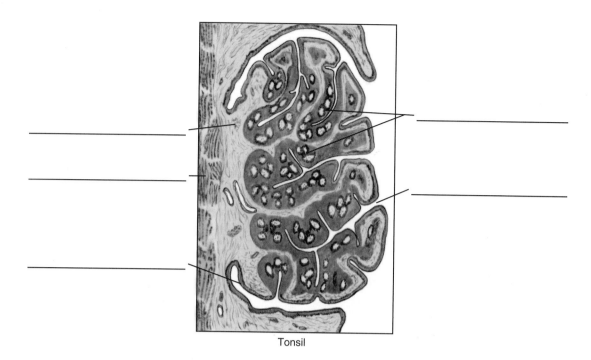

Tonsil

22. Figure 11-20

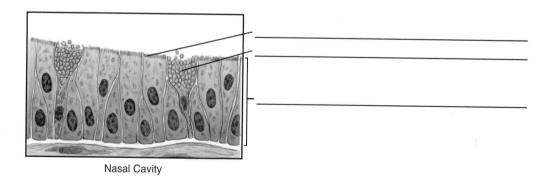

Nasal Cavity

Chapter 12: Enamel

23. Figure 12-6

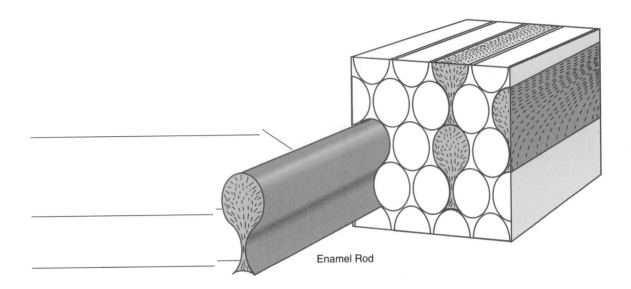

Enamel Rod

Chapter 13: Dentin and Pulp

24. Figures 13-11 and 13-16 combined

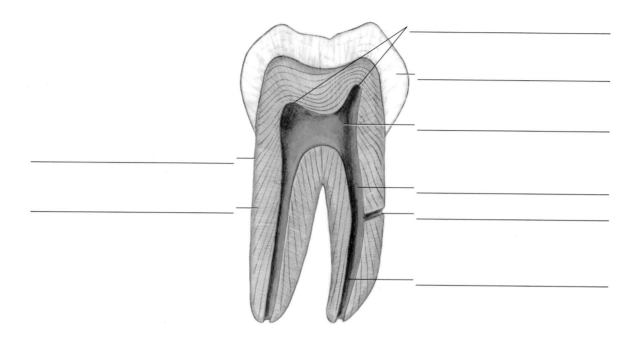

Chapter 14: Periodontium

25. Figure 14-1

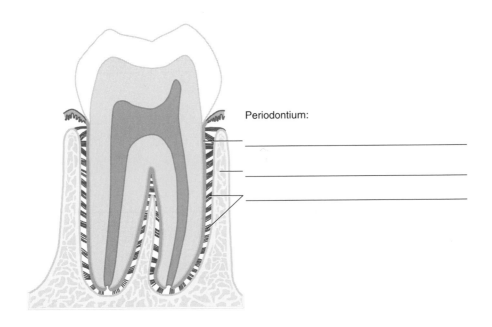

Periodontium:

_____

_____

_____

26. Figure 14-2

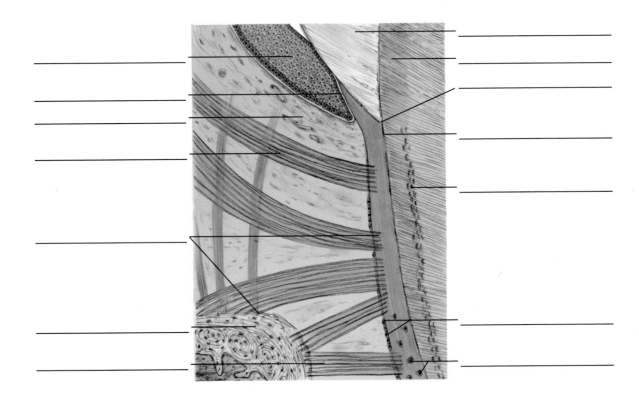

27. Figure 14-14

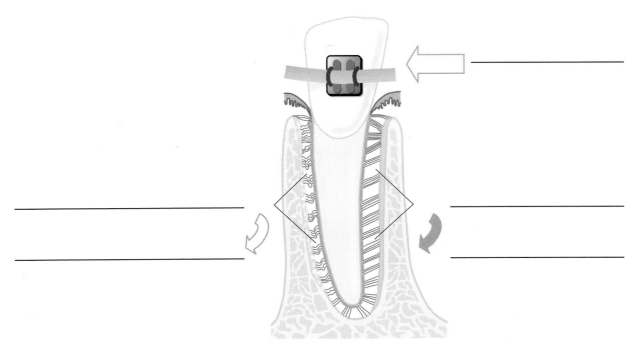

Orthodontic Tooth Movement

28. Figure 14-27

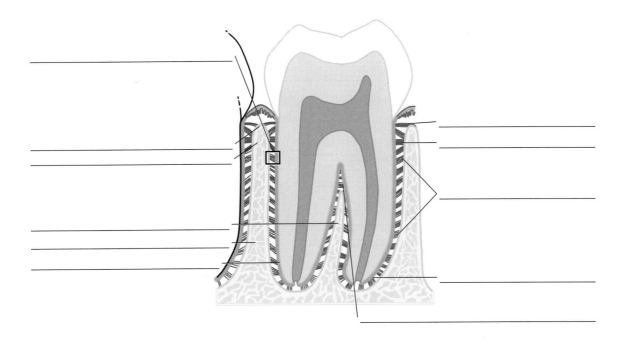

29. Figure 14-31

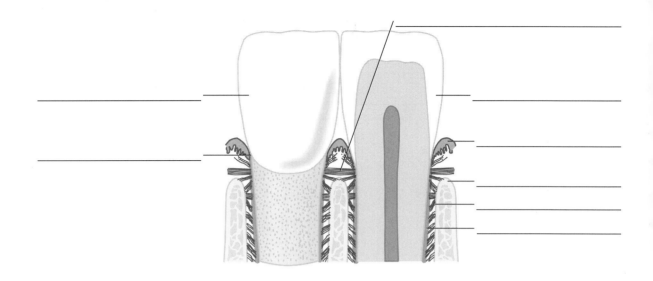

30. Figure 14-32

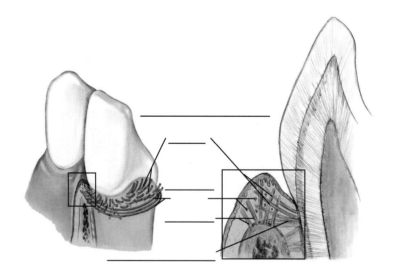

Unit IV: Dental Anatomy

Chapter 15: Overview of Dentitions

1. Figure 15-1

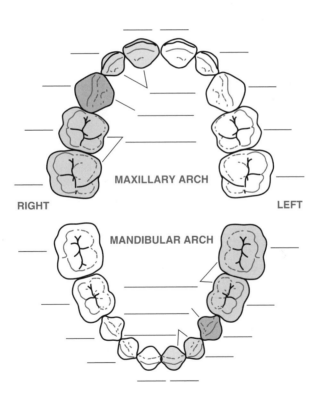

2. Figure 15-2

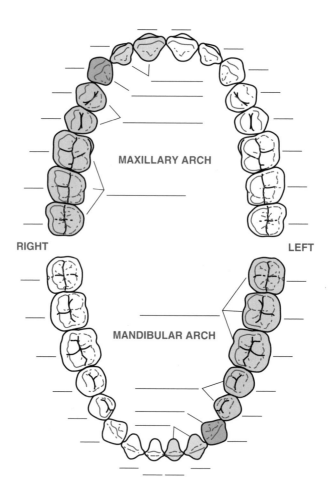

3. Figure 15-5

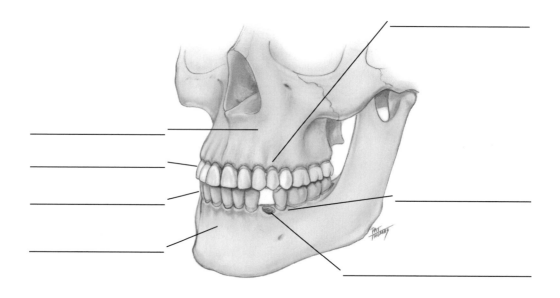

4. Figure 15-6

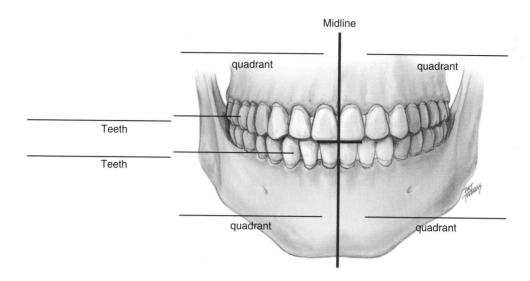

5. Figure 15-7

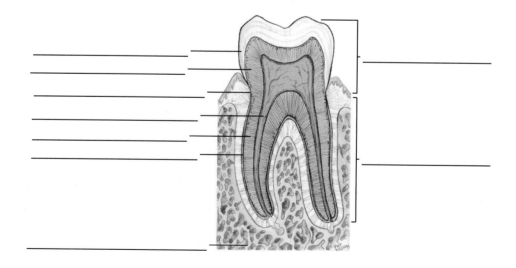

6. Figure 15-8

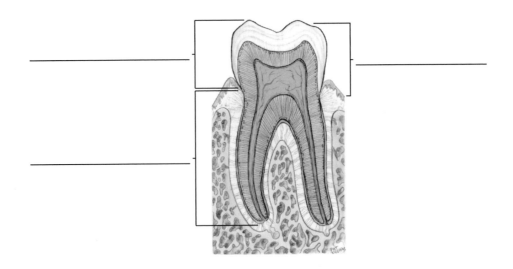

7. Figure 15-9

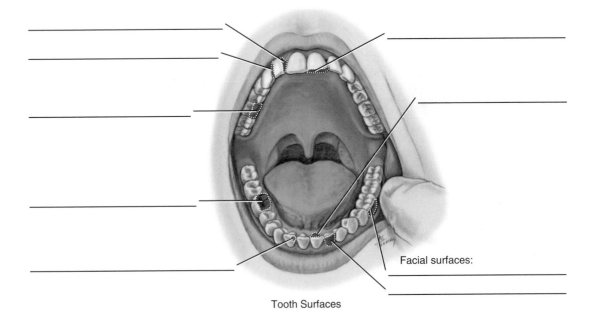

Facial surfaces:

Tooth Surfaces

8. Figure 15-12

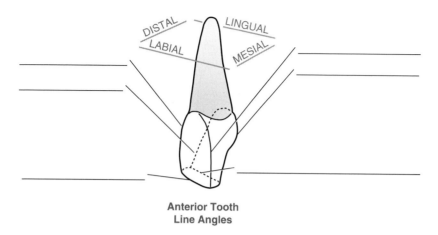

**Anterior Tooth
Line Angles**

9. Figure 15-12

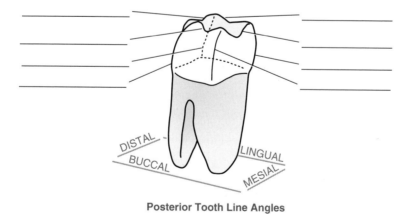

Posterior Tooth Line Angles

10. Figure 15-14

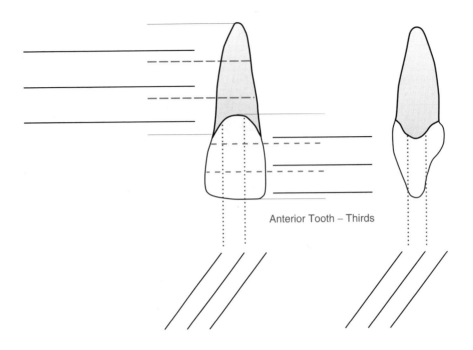

Anterior Tooth – Thirds

11. Figure 15-14

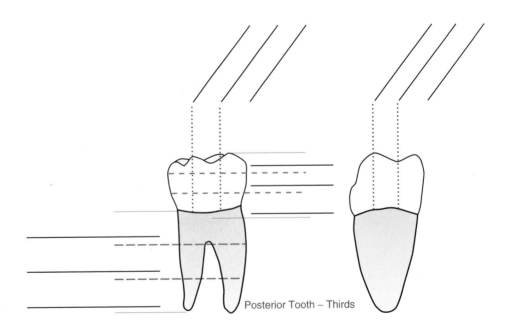

Posterior Tooth – Thirds

Chapter 16: Permanent Anterior Teeth

12. Figure 16-7

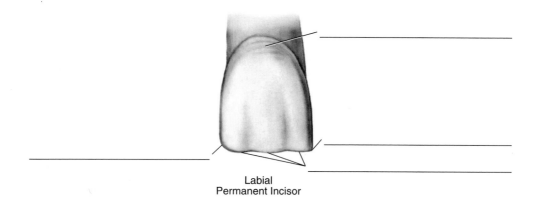

Labial
Permanent Incisor

13. Figure 16-7

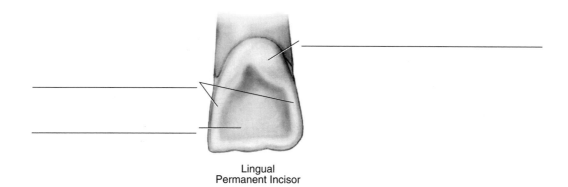

Lingual
Permanent Incisor

14. Figure 16-7

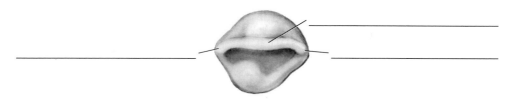

Incisal
Permanent Incisor

15. Figure 16-23

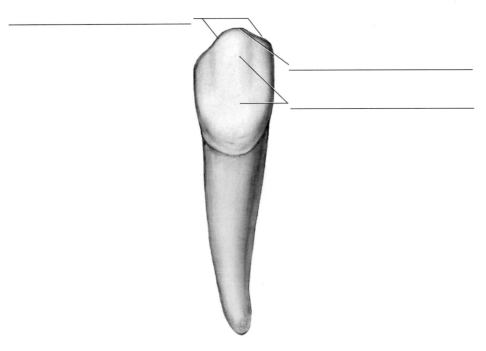

Labial View
Permanent Mandibular Right Canine

16. Figure 16-24

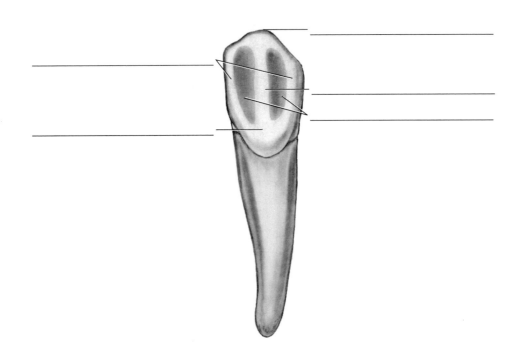

Lingual View
Permanent Mandibular Right Canine

17.   Figure 16-28

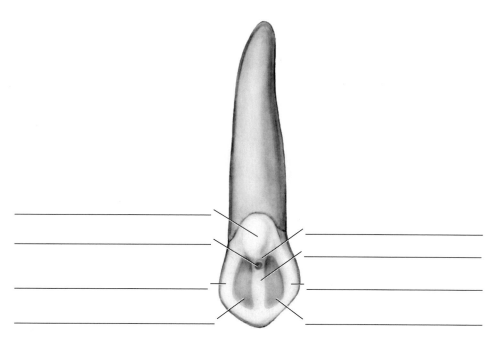

Permanent Maxillary Right Canine

Chapter 17: Permanent Posterior Teeth

18. Figure 17-2

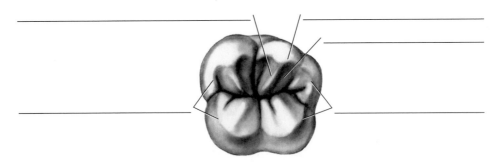

Permanent Posterior Tooth

19. Figure 17-4

Developmental grooves:

Permanent Posterior Tooth

20. Figure 17-13

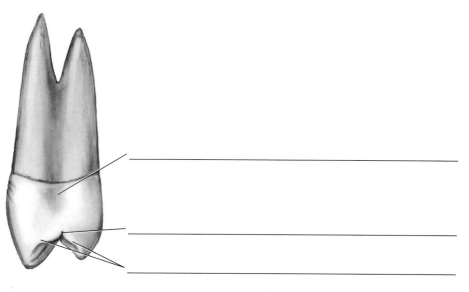

Permanent Maxillary Right First Premolar – Mesial View

21. Figure 17-14

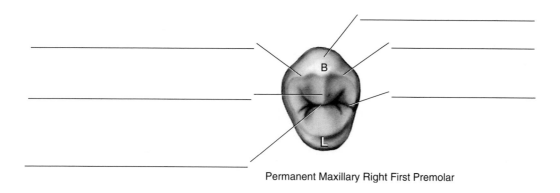

Permanent Maxillary Right First Premolar

22. Figure 17-15

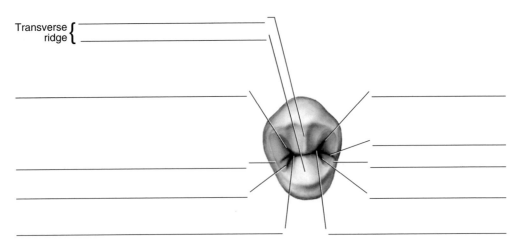

Permanent Maxillary Right First Premolar

23. Figure 17-34

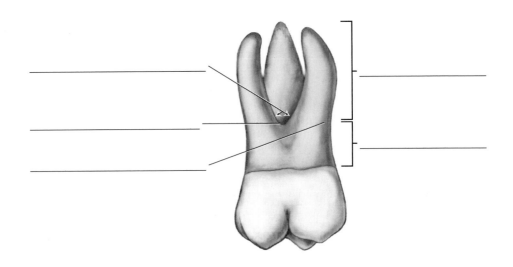

24. Figure 17-34

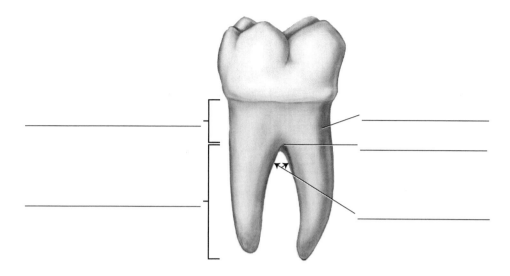

25. Figure 17-40

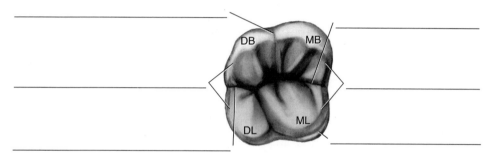

Permanent Maxillary Right First Molar

26. Figure 17-41

Central groove

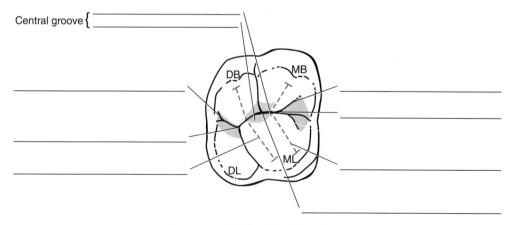

Permanent Maxillary Right First Molar

27. Figure 17-52

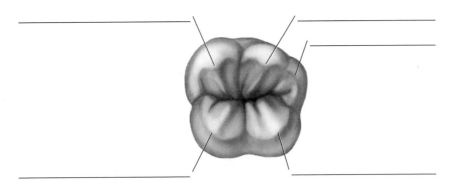

Permanent Mandibular Right First Molar

28. Figure 17-53

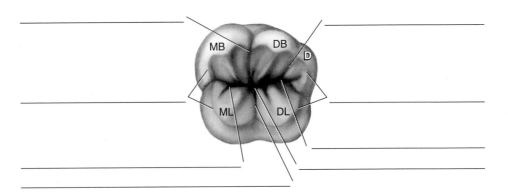

Permanent Mandibular Right First Molar

29. Figure 17-58

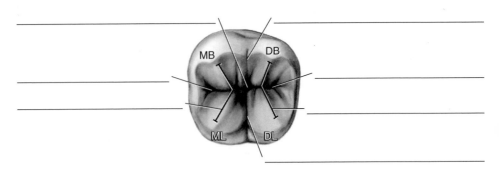

Permanent Mandibular Right Second Molar

Chapter 19: Temporomandibular Joint

30. Figure 19-1

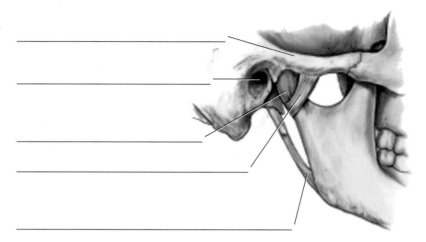

Temporomandibular Joint

31. Figure 19-4

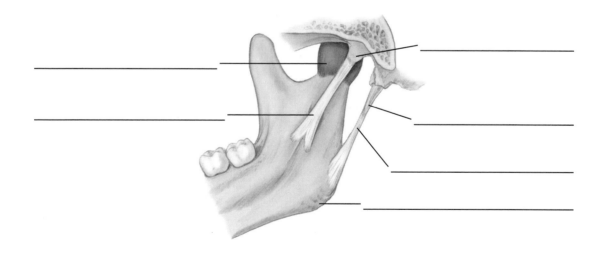

32.   Figure 19-5

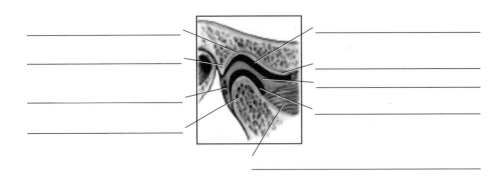

Chapter 20: Occlusion

33. Figure 20-2

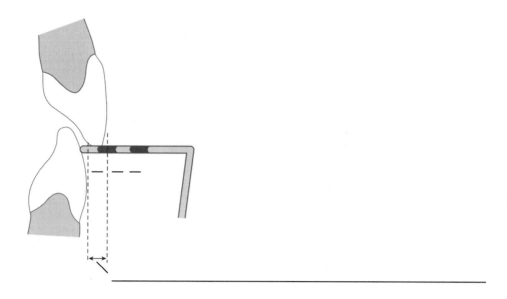

34. Figure 20-2

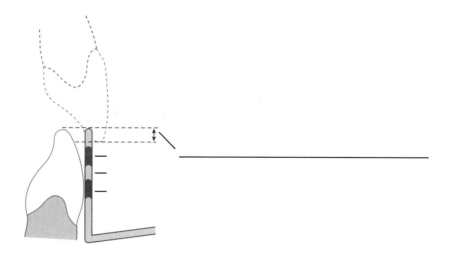

35. Figure 20-20

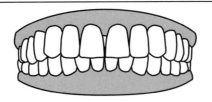

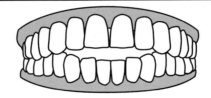

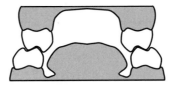

Posterior (bilateral)

Glossary

Exercises

Unit I: Introduction to Dental Structures

Crossword

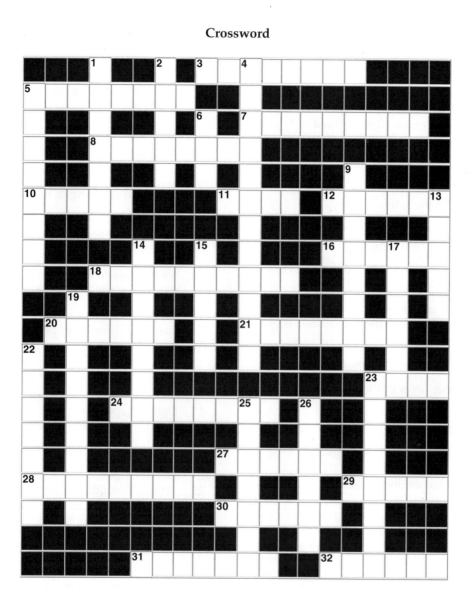

Across:

3 Vertical groove on the midline of the upper lip, extending downward from the nasal septum to the tubercle of the upper lip.

5 Bony process or projection at the anterior border of the mandibular ramus.

7 Small yellowish elevations or spots on the mucosa resulting from deeper deposits of sebum from trapped or misplaced sebaceous glands.

8 Portion of the bone of the maxilla or mandible that supports the teeth.

10 Nostrils of the nose.

11 Main feature of the nasal region of the face is this external feature.

12 Describes structures or facial surfaces of a tooth close to the inner cheek.

16 Alveolar bone between two neighboring teeth which is considered interdental.

18 This part of the face has many structures within it, such as the lips and oral cavity.

20 Hard inner layer of the crown of a tooth overlying the pulp.

21 Socket of the tooth.

23 White ridge of raised keratinized epithelial tissue or linea on the buccal mucosa that extends horizontally at the level where the teeth occlude.

24 Lower jawbone.

27 Hard outer layer of the crown of a tooth.

28 Normal variation in bone growths noted usually on the facial surface of the alveolar process of the maxilla.

29 Bony socket that contains the eyeball and all its supporting structures.

30 Space facing the sulcular gingiva.

31 Bony projection off the posterior and superior border of the mandibular ramus.

32 Voice box in the midline of neck, composed of cartilages.

Down:

1 Opening from the pulp at the apex of the tooth.

2 White ridge of raised keratinized epithelial tissue or linea on the buccal mucosa that extends horizontally at the level where the teeth occlude.

4 Region of the face located both inferior to the orbital region and lateral to the nasal region.

5 Outermost layer of the root of a tooth.

6 Winglike cartilaginous structure bounding the nares laterally.

9 Midline thickening of the upper lip.

13 Tissue fluid that drains from the surrounding region into the lymphatic vessels.

14 Small elevated structures of specialized mucosa on the tongue.

15 Small pitlike depression located where the sulcus terminalis points backward toward the pharynx.

17 Nonencapsulated masses of lymphoid tissue.

19 Darker appearance or zone of the lips compared with the surrounding skin.

22 Anterior teeth that also are the third teeth from the midline in each quadrant.

23 Type of teeth that includes incisors and canines at the front of the oral cavity.

25 Describes structures or tooth surfaces closest to the tongue.

26 Midline fold of tissue between the ventral surface of the tongue and the floor of the mouth.

Words to Find

Ala	Infraorbital	Nose	Submandibular
Angle	Labiomental	Orbit	Submental
Apex	Larynx	Parathyroid	Sulcus
Articulating	Lymph	Parotid	Symphysis
Buccal	Mandible	Philtrum	Temporomandibular
Commissure	Masseter	Proportions	Thyroid
Condyle	Mental	Ramus	Tubercle
Coronoid	Naris	Root	Vermilion
Frontal	Nasal	Sternocleidomastoid	Zygomatic
Hyoid	Nasolabial	Sublingual	

Word Search, Puzzle 1

```
L A R Y N X S K P R O P O R T I O N S I
S R D O G Z H L A T N O R F T O O R D R
I Y A I R E L C R E B U T S Y L W I A Y
S S E L O D I O R Y H T A R A P O L L D
Y S L A U Y H N O S E H Q L O T U A I E
H I Y T G B H P C U S P A A S B T O R S
P R D N E J I I M U Y I L A I I R U U B
M A N E N W T D B Y B A M D B Y S C L M
Y N O M B A J L N A L O N R H S L A Q A
S H C B M A I E L A D A O T I U B V L S
C J U O N N F O L I M A L M S I G A R S
C I G G G K S M E B R O M N O X T B V E
T Y L U E A T L U F I O R M B N E X B T
Z E A Z N N C S N L C D E O E U P P J E
L L V F K O U I U A A N N M P A C X A R
M D I O N O R O C M T S B A R M Y C Y R
A M U R T L I H P A A U A O M I E M A L
P I E A X Q M E L I S R T N J A N T U L
E T C Z E R A H A R T I C U L A T I N G
S N O I L I M R E V D T I B R O G P Z V
```

Words to Find

Alveolar	Foliate	Mucogingival	Raphe
Alveolus	Fordyces	Mucosa	Retromolar
Anterior	Fornix	Nasopharynx	Submandibular
Caruncle	Fungiform	Oropharynx	Taste
Cecum	Gingiva	Parotid	Terminalis
Dorsal	Incisors	Periodontal	Tonsil
Exostoses	Labial	Permanent	Torus
Facial	Lingual	Posterior	Tuberosity
Fauces	Mastication	Premolars	Uvula
Faucial	Melanin	Primary	Ventral
Filiform	Molars	Pterygomandibular	Vestibules
Fimbriata	Mucobuccal	Pulp	

Word Search, Puzzle 2

```
T  S  R  O  S  I  C  N  I  F  P  R  I  M  A  R  Y  F  V  T
S  L  D  E  G  N  L  M  I  L  V  S  A  Q  R  R  R  O  E  O
R  H  A  G  L  A  O  M  R  E  A  S  U  O  W  A  A  L  N  N
A  N  O  V  I  C  B  I  S  O  O  U  I  L  L  L  P  I  T  S
L  Y  U  B  I  R  N  T  T  C  F  R  G  U  O  O  H  A  R  I
O  Y  A  L  I  G  I  U  U  A  E  I  B  N  U  E  E  T  A  L
M  L  T  A  A  B  N  M  R  T  C  I  L  X  I  V  V  E  L  S
E  X  T  I  U  C  L  I  N  A  D  I  W  I  S  L  U  L  I  O
R  A  N  L  S  A  C  A  G  N  C  N  T  U  F  A  J  L  A  L
P  T  E  Y  I  O  D  U  A  O  A  E  B  S  A  T  A  S  A  R
Z  S  N  C  R  O  R  M  B  S  C  M  C  W  A  N  X  T  A  M
F  R  U  E  R  A  O  E  O  O  A  U  E  U  I  M  N  L  R  Y
P  A  O  S  N  G  H  P  B  N  C  X  M  M  M  O  O  O  F  R
F  G  A  I  Y  A  H  P  D  U  O  U  R  U  D  M  F  O  P  M
F  L  I  R  R  A  M  I  O  S  T  E  M  O  O  I  R  A  F  E
W  A  E  N  R  E  B  R  T  R  T  S  I  R  G  D  R  O  A  L
F  T  U  Y  G  U  T  O  E  A  O  R  T  N  Y  O  R  P  C  A
P  A  N  C  L  I  S  S  S  P  E  E  U  C  T  N  U  E  I  N
O  X  T  A  E  E  V  T  O  P  R  F  E  I  I  L  N  F  A  I
T  O  R  U  S  S  E  A  T  P  H  S  D  X  P  I  J  H  L  N
```

Unit II: Dental Embryology

Crossword, Puzzle 1

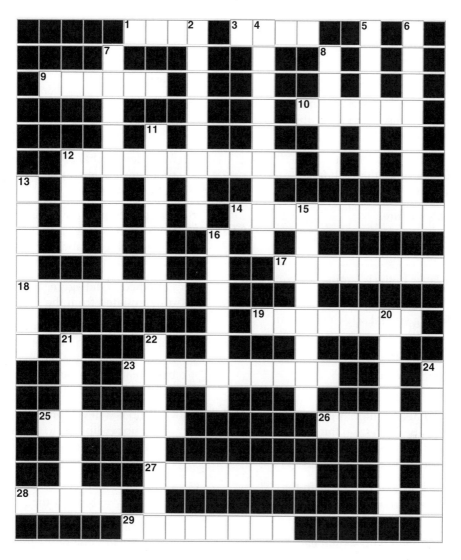

Across:

1 Circular plate of bilayered cells developed from the blastocyst.

3 Depressions in the center of each nasal placode that evolve into the nasal cavities.

9 During prenatal development, the elimination of this between two adjacent swellings occurs during fusion.

10 Type of tube formed when the neural folds meet and fuse superior to the neural groove.

12 Cells that differentiate from preameloblasts and that will form enamel during amelogenesis.

14 Form of a structure.

17 Embryonic layer located between the ectoderm and endoderm.

18 Superior layer in the bilaminar disc.

19 Areas of ectoderm found at the location of developing special sense organs on the embryo.

23 The embryonic disc with three distinct layers: ectoderm, mesoderm, and endoderm.

25 Fused internal and inferior growth (intermaxillary type) from the paired medial nasal processes on the inside of the stomodeum of the embryo.

26 Tail end of a structure, such as in the trilaminar embryonic disc.

27 The primitive streak causes the disc to a right half and left half, so that each half mirrors the other half of the embryo.

28 Structure of the fetal period of prenatal development derived from the enlarged embryo.

29 Process during prenatal development when individual cell division or mitosis converts a zygote to a blastocyst.

Down:

2 Head end of a structure such as in the trilaminar embryonic disc.

4 Process by which the action of one group of cells on another leads to the establishment of the developmental pathway in the responding tissue.

5 Structure derived from the implanted blastocyst.

6 Posterior _____ that develops from the fourth branchial arches and marks the development of the future epiglottis.

7 Birth defects that are developmental problems evident at birth are _____ malformations.

8 Specialized group of cells developed from neuroectoderm that migrate from the neural folds and disperse to specific sites within the mesenchyme.

11 Paired cuboidal aggregates of cells differentiated from the mesoderm.

12 Branchial apparatus (**brang**-ke-al ap-pah-**ra** tis) Group of structures that includes each branchial _____, branchial grooves and membranes, and the pharyngeal pouches.

13 Cleft lip is a developmental disturbance of the upper lip due to failure of fusion of the maxillary processes with the medial nasal _____.

15 Processes that occur from the start of pregnancy to birth of the child.

16 Membrane at the caudal end of the embryo that is the location of the future anus.

20 Layer in the trilaminar embryonic disc derived from the epiblast layer and lining the stomodeum.

21 Anterior portion of the future digestive tract or primitive pharynx that forms the oropharynx.

22 Embryonic membrane that disintegrates, bringing the nasal and oral cavities into communication.

24 Process occurring to the embryo by which places the tissues in their proper positions for further embryonic development.

Crossword, Puzzle 2

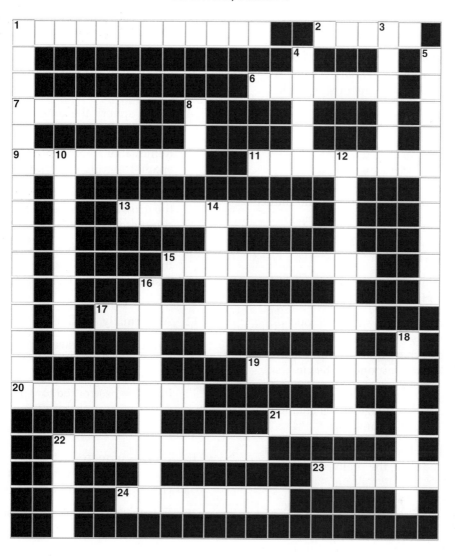

Across:

1 Groove that extends from the medial corner of the eye to the nasal cavity.

2 Developmental disturbance due to failure of fusion of the palatal shelves with the primary palate or with each other.

6 Two processes derived from the maxillary processes during prenatal development.

7 Portion of the cervical loop that functions to shape the root(s) and induce dentin formation in the root area.

9 Cementum matrix laid down by cementoblasts.

11 Circular plate of bilayered cells developed from the blastocyst.

13 Process by which the action of one group of cells on another that leads to the establishment of the developmental pathway in the responding tissue.

15 Layered formation of a firm or hard tissue such as cartilage, bone, enamel, dentin, and cementum.

17 Process by which the sperm penetrates the ovum during the preimplantation period.

19 Photographic analysis of a person's chromosomes.

20 Primitive mouth, which initially appears as a shallow depression in the embryonic surface.

21 Cap or bell shaped portion of the tooth germ that produces enamel.

22 Structure during prenatal development consisting of trophoblast cells and an inner mass of cells that develop into the embryo.

23 Substance in connective tissue composed of intercellular substance and fibers or extracellular substance that is partially calcified and serves as a framework for later calcification.

24 Layer in the trilaminar embryonic disc derived from the hypoblast layer.

Down:

1 Permanent teeth without primary predecessors, namely the molars.

3 A dental developmental disturbance in which two adjacent tooth germs unite, forming a large tooth.

4 Small, spherical enamel projection on the tooth surface.

5 Removal of a hard tissue such as bone, enamel, dentin, or cementum.

8 Second stage of tooth development with the growth of the dental lamina into the ectomesenchyme.

10 Groups of epithelial cells of _____ in the periodontal ligament after the disintegration of Hertwig's epithelial root sheath.

12 Abnormally small teeth.

14 Pair of posterior swellings formed from the third and fourth branchial arches, which overgrow the second arches to form the base of the tongue.

16 Dentin matrix laid down by apposition by the odontoblasts.

18 Process of reproductive cell production that ensures the correct number of chromosomes for the future embryo.

22 Fourth stage of odontogenesis, in which differentiation occurs to its furthest extent.

Words to Find

Amniocentesis	Ectoderm	Induction	Primordium
Bilaminar	Embryo	Karyotype	Somites
Blastocyst	Endoderm	Maturation	Symmetry
Caudal	Epiblast	Meiosis	Teratogens
Cephalic	Fertilization	Mesoderm	Trilaminar
Cleavage	Fetus	Mitosis	Zygote
Cloacal	Folding	Morphology	
Congenital	Fusion	Neuroectoderm	
Disc	Hypoblast	Prenatal	

Word Search, Puzzle 1

```
Q  F  E  V  U  D  C  L  L  S  F  D  C  L  E  A  V  A  G  E
A  B  P  T  X  S  F  L  M  E  S  O  D  E  R  M  S  M  L  S
Q  E  I  R  S  Y  M  M  E  T  R  Y  B  I  H  N  R  A  I  N
C  C  B  I  B  L  A  S  T  O  C  Y  S  T  E  E  T  S  O  S
L  T  L  L  M  I  T  O  S  I  S  G  R  G  D  I  E  I  U  W
O  O  A  A  W  R  C  L  V  S  J  S  O  O  N  T  T  T  E  P
A  D  S  M  Y  J  A  N  I  A  E  T  T  E  N  C  E  T  R  H
C  E  T  I  W  D  G  S  G  T  A  C  G  E  U  F  F  D  P  Z
A  R  M  N  U  B  O  D  I  R  E  N  C  D  E  P  E  Q  R  C
L  M  E  A  C  I  L  M  E  O  O  O  N  C  H  I  R  J  E  R
M  G  C  R  E  U  O  T  R  C  I  I  P  M  Y  D  T  K  N  O
J  A  B  M  F  S  Y  U  C  N  H  K  R  O  P  S  I  U  A  E
F  C  T  I  X  O  E  W  M  U  U  A  I  R  O  A  L  E  T  M
U  E  M  U  L  N  L  A  J  H  R  R  M  P  B  B  I  N  A  B
S  P  D  R  R  A  Z  D  O  Q  I  Y  O  H  L  X  Z  D  L  R
I  H  J  H  A  A  M  Y  I  U  Y  O  R  O  A  S  A  O  U  Y
O  A  D  G  L  Z  T  I  G  N  U  T  D  L  S  F  T  D  H  O
N  L  J  I  R  D  L  I  N  O  G  Y  I  O  T  F  I  E  Z  T
K  I  U  J  S  S  V  F  O  A  T  P  U  G  C  L  O  R  Q  B
B  C  Q  T  O  C  K  O  H  N  R  E  M  Y  L  K  N  M  X  V
```

Words to Find

Apposition	Ectomesenchyme	Membrane	Preameloblasts
Bell	Fusion	Microdontia	Predentin
Bud	Gemination	Morphogenesis	Repolarization
Cementoblasts	Induction	Nonsuccedaneous	Resorption
Cementocytes	Initiation	Odontoblasts	Sheath
Cementoid	Macrodontia	Odontoclasts	Succedaneous
Dilaceration	Malassez	Organ	Supernumerary
Ectoderm	Matrix	Pearl	

Word Search, Puzzle 2

```
W  C  X  O  O  X  X  L  C  E  M  E  N  T  O  C  Y  T  E  S
M  M  A  L  A  S  S  E  Z  E  N  N  N  N  S  N  S  S  V  X
I  B  S  F  U  S  I  O  N  I  O  O  O  I  O  T  U  K  I  E
C  R  E  S  Y  G  K  A  T  I  I  I  S  I  S  O  Y  R  O  S
R  Z  X  L  P  J  R  N  T  T  E  T  A  E  F  T  O  T  O
O  F  P  Q  L  B  E  A  I  A  N  A  L  N  O  A  S  S  B  L
D  C  C  L  M  D  N  S  I  E  Z  B  A  E  M  N  A  X  R  N
O  E  Z  E  E  I  O  T  G  I  O  D  V  C  H  L  W  A  A  S
N  M  M  R  M  P  I  O  R  L  E  E  N  T  B  F  E  G  O  U
T  E  P  E  P  N  H  A  E  C  Z  O  A  O  M  P  R  I  D  P
I  N  G  A  I  P  L  M  C  G  I  E  T  M  A  O  R  N  O  E
A  T  D  D  R  O  A  U  Q  T  H  N  K  E  C  C  E  D  N  R
R  O  U  O  P  E  S  J  A  S  O  O  B  S  R  E  S  U  T  N
O  B  M  E  R  N  L  R  H  D  E  H  M  E  O  M  O  C  O  U
E  L  R  P  O  Q  E  S  O  T  Y  Q  R  N  D  E  R  T  C  M
K  A  W  N  E  C  E  B  M  Q  N  D  M  C  O  N  P  I  L  E
I  S  R  C  A  E  C  T  O  D  E  R  M  H  N  T  T  O  A  R
R  T  U  L  N  E  Q  L  J  M  D  F  B  Y  T  O  I  N  S  A
A  S  I  S  D  P  B  I  O  Y  P  C  U  M  I  I  O  F  T  R
C  D  J  A  S  U  W  R  V  E  E  R  T  E  A  D  N  H  S  Y
```

Unit III: Dental Histology

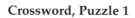

Crossword, Puzzle 1

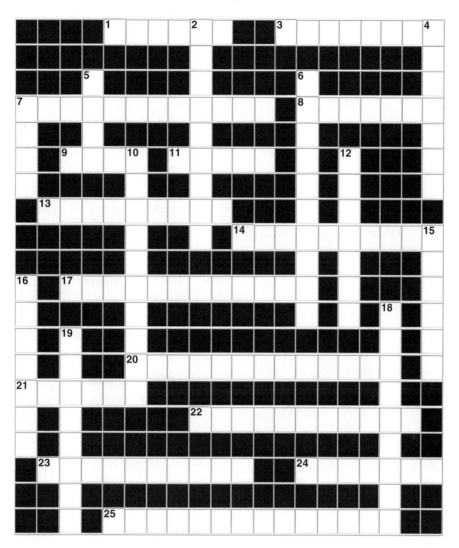

Across:

1 Group of organs functioning together.

3 Closely apposed sheets of bone tissue in compact bone.

7 Organelles associated with manufacture of ATP.

8 Largest, densest, and most conspicuous organelle in the cell.

9 Smallest unit of organization in the body.

11 Somewhat independent body part that performs a specific function or functions and that is formed from tissues.

13 Chief nucleoprotein in the nondividing nucleoplasm.

14 White blood cell that increases in numbers during an immune response.

17 Three-dimensional system of support within the cell.

20 Type of intermediate filament that has a major role in intercellular junctions.

21 Structure formed by the grouping of cells with similar characteristics of shape and function.

22 Immature connective tissue formed during initial repair.

23 Two filamentous daughter chromosomes joined at a centromere during cell division.

24 Specialized connective tissue composed of fat, little matrix, and adipocytes.

25 Along with calcium, the main inorganic crystal in enamel, bone, dentin, and cementum.

Down:

2 Superficial layers of the skin.

4 Type of protein fiber in connective tissue composed of microfilaments.

5 Rigid connective tissue.

6 Metabolically inert substances or transient structures within the cell.

7 White blood cell that is similar to the basophil because it is also involved in allergic responses.

10 Second most common white blood cell in the blood, involved in the immune response.

12 Portion of cell division that occurs in phases and results in two daughter cells that are identical to the parent cell.

15 Small space that surrounds the chondrocyte or osteocyte within the cartilage matrix or bone, respectively.

16 Type of intermediate protein filament that is found in calloused epithelial tissues and consists of an opaque waterproof substance.

18 Intercellular junction between cells.

19 White blood cell that contains granules of histamine and heparin.

Crossword, Puzzle 2

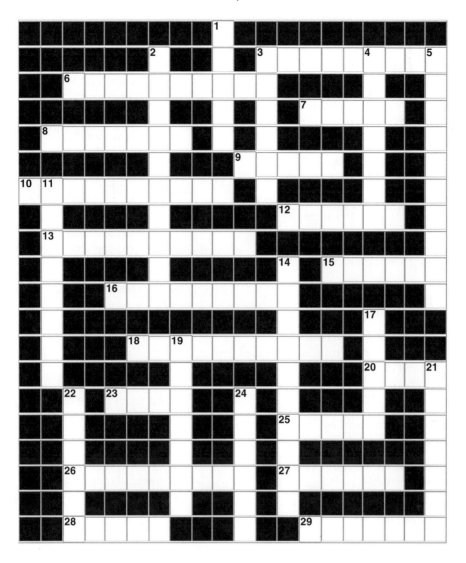

Across:

3 Tissue deep to the oral mucosa, composed of loose connective tissue.

6 Joined matrix pieces forming a lattice in cancellous bone.

7 Tissue fluid that drains from the surrounding region into the lymphatic vessels.

8 Initially formed bone matrix.

9 In a salivary gland, a central opening where the saliva is deposited into a duct after being produced by the secretory cells.

10 Mature osteoblasts entrapped in bone matrix.

12 Cells in respiratory mucosa that produce mucus that keeps this mucosa moist.

13 Network of vssels that collect and transport lymph, linking lymph nodes throughout most of the body.

15 Cavities with hard tooth tissue loss resulting from demineralization of the tooth due to acid produced by cariogenic bacteria.

16 Blood cell fragments that function in the clotting mechanism.

18 Dense connective tissue layer on the outer portion of bone.

20 Extensions or ridges of the epithelium into the connective tissue as they appear on histological section.

23 Passageway that allows a glandular secretion to be emptied directly into the location where the secretion is to be used.

25 Large inner portions of certain glands.

26 Dense connective tissue in the dermis and lamina propria.

27 Secretion from salivary glands that lubricates and cleanses the oral cavity and helps in digestion.

28 Bundle of neural processes outside the central nervous system.

29 Localized macules of pigmentation.

Down:

1 Depression on one side of the lymph node.

2 Grooves noted on some teeth in the oral cavity, associated with the lines of Retzius in enamel.

3 Connective tissue that helps divide the inner portion of certain glands.

4 Connective tissue that surrounds the outer portion of the entire gland or lesion.

5 Cells that differentiate from preameloblasts and that will form enamel during amelogenesis.

11 Epithelium that stands away from the tooth, creating a gingival sulcus.

14 Cell that functions in resorption of bone.

17 Nostril of the nose.

19 Incremental lines of _____ in preparations of mature enamel.

21 Hard tooth tissue loss through chemical means (acid), not involving bacteria.

22 Functional cellular component of the nervous system.

24 Extracellular substance that is partially calcified and serves as a framework for later calcification.

Crossword, Puzzle 3

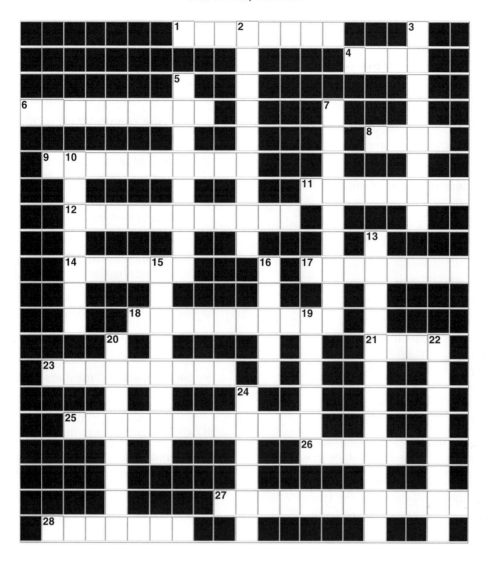

Across:

1 Inflammation of the pulp.

4 Soft innermost connective tissue in both the crown and root of the tooth.

6 Hard tooth tissue loss by from tooth to tooth contact from mastication or parafunctional habits.

8 The crystalline structural unit of enamel.

9 Layered formation of a firm or hard tissue such as enamel, dentin, and cementum.

11 Surrounds the teeth and supports and attaches the teeth to the bony surface of the alveoli.

12 Incremental lines or bands of von Ebner in mature dentin.

14 Opening or foramen from the pulp at the apex of the tooth.

17 Socket of the tooth.

18 Cancellous bone that is located between the alveolar bone proper and the plates of cortical bone.

21 Adjoining imbrication lines in dentin that demonstrate a disturbance in body metabolism.

23 Extra openings located on the lateral portions of the roots of some teeth.

25 Apposition of enamel matrix by ameloblasts.

26 Microscopic feature in mature enamel consisting of small dark brushes with their bases near the dentinoenamel junction.

27 Layer of dentin around the outer pulpal wall.

28 Portion of the tooth that contains the mass of pulp.

Down:

2 Dentin matrix laid down by apposition by the odontoblasts.

3 Microscopic feature present in mature enamel consisting of short dentinal tubules near the dentinoenamel junction.

5 Plates of compact bone on the facial and lingual surfaces of the alveolar bone.

7 Portion of the pulp located in the root area of the tooth.

10 Dentin formed in a tooth before the completion of the apical foramen.

13 Supporting hard and soft dental tissues between and including portions of the tooth and the alveolar bone.

15 Hard tooth tissue loss by friction from toothbrushing and/or toothpaste.

16 There is _____ within the dentinal tubule in dentin.

19 Smooth, stained microscopic lines noted in cartilage, bone, and cementum due to apposition occurring in these tissues.

20 Outermost layer of the root of a tooth.

22 Accentuated incremental line of Retzius in enamel or contour line of Owen in dentin that results from birth process.

24 Hard inner layer of the crown of a tooth overlying the pulp.

Words to Find

Cell	Endocytosis	Microfilaments	Prophase
Centromere	Exocytosis	Microtubules	Ribosomes
Centrosome	Hemidesmosome	Mitochondria	System
Chromatids	Histology	Mitosis	Telophase
Chromatin	Inclusions	Nucleolus	Tissue
Chromosomes	Interphase	Nucleoplasm	Tonofilaments
Cytoplasm	Keratin	Nucleus	Vacuoles
Cytoskeleton	Lysosomes	Organ	
Desmosome	Metaphase	Phagocytosis	

Word Search, Puzzle 1

```
M  I  M  E  K  W  Q  Q  P  H  A  G  O  C  Y  T  O  S  I  S
I  J  E  X  K  U  N  W  E  E  M  S  S  S  S  S  S  E  A  A
T  G  T  D  B  E  U  U  S  S  I  E  I  D  S  T  S  E  I  E
O  D  A  I  I  K  S  A  A  S  M  S  I  U  N  A  Q  R  M  S
S  M  P  K  K  S  H  L  O  O  O  T  L  E  H  S  D  O  E  M
I  M  H  L  I  P  P  T  S  T  A  O  M  P  E  N  S  L  S  J
S  J  A  T  O  O  Y  O  Y  M  E  A  O  M  O  O  O  A  E  S
M  I  S  L  T  C  M  C  O  L  L  R  O  H  R  U  L  M  T  N
I  N  E  Y  O  O  O  R  C  I  P  S  C  T  C  P  O  N  I  S
C  T  C  X  R  D  H  U  F  Y  O  O  N  A  O  S  E  T  N  V
R  E  E  H  N  C  N  O  X  M  T  E  V  E  O  M  A  O  W  E
O  R  C  E  P  H  R  G  S  I  C  O  L  M  A  R  I  L  R  C
T  P  I  C  F  C  I  E  M  N  U  C  S  L  E  S  L  E  T  H
U  H  G  B  I  N  D  S  A  U  U  E  I  K  U  L  M  N  Z  R
B  A  S  M  O  I  U  G  T  N  D  F  I  L  E  O  S  S  T  O
U  S  M  S  M  S  R  C  B  O  O  L  C  C  R  L  F  Y  O  M
L  E  R  E  W  O  O  M  L  N  L  N  R  T  H  P  E  S  A  A
E  V  H  O  O  Q  Z  M  O  E  I  O  N  M  B  N  H  T  D  T
S  D  D  Z  D  I  Q  T  E  C  U  E  G  R  T  H  J  E  O  I
L  Y  S  O  S  O  M  E  S  S  C  S  X  Y  Z  N  V  M  O  N
```

Words to Find

Adipose	Collagen	Fibroblast	Keratin
Appositional	Dermis	Granulation	Lacuna
Basophil	Elastic	Haversian	Lamellae
Bone	Endosteum	Hemidesmosomes	Lymphocyte
Canaliculi	Endothelium	Hydroxyapatite	Macrophage
Cartilage	Eosinophil	Immunogen	Mast
Chondroblasts	Epidermis	Immunoglobulin	
Chondrocytes	Epithelium	Interstitial	

Word Search, Puzzle 2

```
N  E  S  J  X  J  V  B  O  N  E  C  A  R  T  I  L  A  G  E
M  A  S  T  E  P  I  T  H  E  L  I  U  M  L  A  C  U  N  A
U  J  E  I  J  C  B  D  L  M  X  B  D  R  O  Z  T  Z  I  C
W  I  L  M  J  H  E  I  U  L  A  M  E  L  L  A  E  L  F  W
I  J  A  M  O  O  I  M  M  U  N  O  G  L  O  B  U  L  I  N
H  Z  S  U  E  N  Q  K  V  M  M  E  P  I  D  E  R  M  I  S
I  C  T  N  A  D  D  E  R  M  I  S  D  R  O  K  X  Y  G  H
T  L  I  O  P  R  C  B  F  O  F  I  B  R  O  B  L  A  S  T
G  D  C  G  P  O  I  I  F  A  M  A  C  R  O  P  H  A  G  E
G  B  G  E  O  C  H  E  M  I  D  E  S  M  O  S  O  M  E  S
E  B  R  N  S  Y  Q  I  W  E  N  D  O  T  H  E  L  I  U  M
O  U  A  H  I  T  W  C  H  O  N  D  R  O  B  L  A  S  T  S
S  B  N  A  T  E  Q  C  P  V  A  J  C  O  L  L  A  G  E  N
I  A  U  V  I  S  J  A  D  I  P  O  S  E  Z  S  V  P  U  C
N  S  L  E  O  Y  G  J  D  S  D  D  R  K  E  R  A  T  I  N
O  O  A  R  N  Q  E  W  U  F  L  Y  M  P  H  O  C  Y  T  E
P  P  T  S  A  W  Z  S  I  N  T  E  R  S  T  I  T  I  A  L
H  H  I  I  L  K  C  U  O  B  I  E  N  D  O  S  T  E  U  M
I  I  O  A  R  F  H  Y  D  R  O  X  Y  A  P  A  T  I  T  E
L  L  N  N  W  J  Q  B  B  I  C  A  N  A  L  I  C  U  L  I
```

Words to Find

Endochondral	Odontoclast	Papillary	Squames
Intramembranous	Ossification	Perichondrium	Submucosa
Matrix	Osteoblasts	Periosteum	Synapse
Monocyte	Osteoclast	Plasma	Tonofilaments
Nerve	Osteocytes	Platelets	Trabeculae
Neuron	Osteoid	Rete	
Neutrophil	Osteons	Reticular	

Word Search, Puzzle 3

```
U S P L A S M A E L L I C O I O H X L Z
B U T F Z M F W P Y R X F Z A T C D N L
J B O Y Y W N D L H W F J R S T I O A X
I M N R V S Y N A P S E F A H O I R S M
V U O E F K F O T J I W L O E T D K U B
P C F T L I B X E S H C T T A N U E A K
L O I I Z N S O L D O W S C O A T W B U
T S L C G T P F E E I O I H W S V T P Z
L A A U V R G W T E P F C H O O S F E G
B C M L O A S S S C I O S I E A E P R X
L T E A S M O P V S D C R T L V O A I N
E R N R T E N L S N K E Y C R N S P C E
W A T G E M B O E R P C O E O Z T I H U
O B S S O B D R I D O T N Z O F E L O T
N E X Q B R R G X N N C W M S B O L N R
E C K U L A P P O O M V K A T V C A D O
U U B A A N K M D A V E C T E K Y R R P
R L R M S O M O D J T P E R O G T Y I H
O A J E T U N K W E A J S I N K E W U I
N E T S S S F K R I C U H X S B S X M L
```

Words to Find

Afferent	Germinal	Lobes	Periodontitis
Capsule	Gingivitis	Lobules	Prickle
Colloid	Goblet	Lumen	Recession
Dentogingival	Goiter	Lymph	Stippling
Duct	Granulation	Masticatory	Sulcular
Efferent	Hilus	Melanin	Sulcus
Endocrine	Hyperkeratinized	Mucogingival	Taste
Exocrine	Junctional	Mucoperiosteum	
Fibroblast	Keratin	Mucosa	
Follicles	Keratohyaline	Nodes	

Word Search, Puzzle 4

```
N O D E S E G V K Y Q K A O S U L C U S
A P C K O N P E H K A U R F E L E I T P
H R O H D D M Z R G E E S N F N Y S Y T
A I L H K O U U D M T R I L I E A M C D
E C L Z L C H D C I I R A L O L R U P G
T K O U I R Y E O O C N A T B B D E N H
A L I T S I P G G O P Y A O I S E I N N
P E D D T N E Y X O H E R L E N L S O T
E S W E A E R E E O B B R L M P B I Z L
R E M N S M K Z T A I L C I P G S S A N
I G A T T U E A M F T I E I O S T V O S
O I S O E D R L P S L E T T E S I I E Z
D N T G I E A V A L U S Z C N G T L W A
O G I I K C T V O N I L E L N A U E S V
N I C N E A I F X G I R C I L B Z O U V
T V A G X P N I A J A N G U O A C L Y M
I I T I V S I M O M J O N L L U P U U N
T T O V F U Z S H N C A M W M A I M Z L
I I R A D L E P B U R M E F F E R E N T
S S Y L X E D Z M G J U N C T I O N A L
```

Words to Find

Abfraction	Erosion	Parathyroid	Sinusitis
Abrasion	Lymphadenopathy	Perikymata	Thyroglossal
Ameloblast	Lymphatics	Ranula	Thyroid
Amelogenesis	Mucocele	Retzius	Thyroxine
Attrition	Mucoserous	Saliva	Tonsils
Caries	Myoepithelial	Secretory	Trabeculae
Demilune	Naris	Septum	Xerostomia

Word Search, Puzzle 5

```
I  B  W  S  T  H  Y  R  O  X  I  N  E  T  T  P  E  Z  P  B
S  A  B  F  R  A  C  T  I  O  N  N  K  F  S  K  Z  E  S  S
L  C  A  R  I  E  S  I  L  H  O  G  X  Z  V  I  A  U  I  A
P  A  R  A  T  H  Y  R  O  I  D  Y  E  U  Y  L  O  S  T  T
F  G  Y  L  S  I  N  U  S  I  T  I  S  H  U  R  E  A  S  N
G  D  Y  W  H  G  I  A  M  P  S  K  T  C  E  N  M  A  O  W
Y  E  D  M  U  U  R  X  L  R  N  A  E  S  E  Y  L  I  A  S
M  M  S  S  U  B  U  M  E  Y  P  B  O  G  K  B  T  D  C  D
U  I  A  E  A  J  C  Y  R  O  A  C  O  I  O  I  S  I  I  S
C  L  L  P  N  Z  W  O  N  R  U  L  R  L  R  V  T  O  U  N
O  U  I  T  I  W  T  E  T  M  E  E  E  T  D  A  R  I  O  C
C  N  V  U  U  E  D  P  E  M  P  M  T  F  H  Y  Z  I  D  L
E  E  A  M  R  A  Q  I  A  U  A  A  R  P  H  T  S  K  Q  F
L  H  T  C  H  U  R  T  Z  U  B  P  M  T  E  O  W  M  M  X
E  G  E  P  Y  G  A  H  R  F  R  Y  U  R  R  U  Q  I  G  W
P  S  M  F  Z  X  N  E  O  Y  L  W  G  E  R  G  D  A  N  T
X  Y  U  B  Z  A  U  L  E  F  X  E  R  O  S  T  O  M  I  A
L  K  N  K  S  F  L  I  C  Q  L  L  E  T  O  N  S  I  L  S
I  E  U  V  W  F  A  A  T  H  Y  R  O  G  L  O  S  S  A  L
P  H  T  B  F  V  N  L  N  A  R  I  S  B  F  W  H  S  U  Q
```

Words to Find

Accessory	Cementoid	Imbrication	Principal
Alveolus	Cementum	Interglobular	Pulp
Apical	Chamber	Intertubular	Pulpitis
Apposition	Circumpulpal	Mantle	Radicular
Arrest	Dentin	Neonatal	Secondary
Attrition	Dentinogenesis	Odontoblasts	Stones
Canaliculi	Edentulous	Owen	Tertiary
Cementicles	Fluid	Periodontium	Trabecular
Cementoblasts	Globular	Peritubular	Tubules
Cementocytes	Hypecementosis	Predentin	
Cementogenesis	Hypersensitivity	Primary	

Word Search, Puzzle 6

```
A T T A T Q M P N T G K O I B S A D C C
R E U L C P A U E R D A W M P T T B E H
R R B V E R N L O A E P E B R O T U M A
E T U E M I T P N B N I N R I N R B E M
S I L O E N L I A E T C H I M E I H N B
T A E L N C E T T C I A Y C A S T Z T E
C R S U T I C I A U N L P A R H I C U R
E Y P S O P E S L L O I E T Y Y O E M C
M P E C I A M E I A G N R I O P N M P E
E E R I D L E V N R E T S O D E K E R M
N R I R K C N E T Z N E E N O C A N E E
T I O C S A T D E R E R N A N E P T D N
I T D U E N O E R A S G S C T M P O E T
C U O M C A G N T D I L I C O E O C N O
L B N P O L E T U I S O T E B N S Y T B
E U T U N I N U B C F B I S L T I T I L
S L I L D C E L U U L U V S A O T E N A
U A U P A U S O L L U L I O S S I S W S
I R M A R L I U A A I A T R T I O Q R T
Y Q X L Y I S S R R D R Y Y S S N E Q S
```

Unit IV: Dental Anatomy

Crossword, Puzzle 1

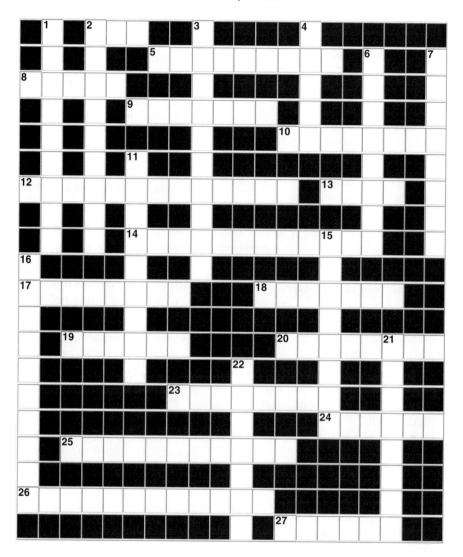

Across:

2 A small lateral incisor crown or third molar crown due to a developmental disturbance of partial microdontia.

5 Natural teeth in the jawbones, consisting of primary and permanent.

8 Mythological creature who at night takes children's shed primary teeth from under their pillows and leaves a sum of cash.

9 Crest of curvature, which is the greatest elevation of the tooth either incisocervically or occlusocervically on a specific surface of the crown.

10 Rounded enamel extensions on the incisal ridge from the labial or lingual views of certain anterior teeth.

12 Tooth designation system using a two digit code.

13 Imaginary line representing the long axis line of a tooth, drawn to bisect cervical line.

14 Crown or root(s) showing angular distortion.

17 Rounded raised borders or ridges on the mesial and distal portions of the lingual surface of anterior teeth and the occlusal table of posterior teeth.

18 Older dental term for canines.

19 Surface of a tooth closest to the midline.

20 Masticatory surface of posterior teeth.

23 Vertically oriented and labially placed bony ridge of alveolar bone noted in the jawbones, especially in the maxilla, near the canine.

24 Surface of the tooth farthest away from the midline.

25 Indentations on the surface of the root(s).

26 Secondary groove that is a shallower, more irregular linear depression and that branches from the developmental grooves on the lingual surface of anterior teeth and the occlusal table on posterior teeth.

27 Division of a crown surface or root into three portions: the crown horizontally and vertically and root horizontally.

Down:

1 Division of each dental arch into two parts, with four quadrants in the entire oral cavity.

2 The second dentition.

3 Portion of root covered by cementum.

4 Shallow, wide depressions on the lingual surface of anterior teeth or on the occlusal table of posterior teeth.

6 Complete displacement of the tooth from the socket due to extensive trauma to the area.

7 Open contact that can exist between the permanent maxillary central incisors.

11 Absence of a single tooth or multiple teeth due to lack of initiation.

15 Unerupted or partially erupted tooth that is positioned against another tooth, bone, or even soft tissue so that complete eruption becomes unlikely.

16 Spaces formed from the curvatures where two teeth in the same arch contact.

21 Division of each dental arch into three portions based on the relationship to the midline.

22 Linear elevation or ridge on the incisal or masticatory surface of permanent incisors when newly erupted.

Crossword, Puzzle 2

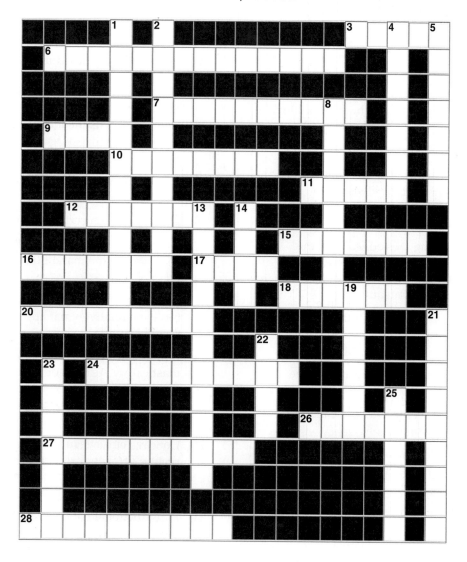

Across:

3   Situation in which the entire posterior quadrant functions during lateral occlusion.

6   Movements of the mandible that are not within the normal motions associated with mastication, speech, or respiratory movements.

7   Moving the lower jaw forward.

9   The _____ of the temporomandibular joint that is located between the temporal bone and condyle of the mandible.

10   Ridge running mesiodistally in the cervical one third of the buccal crown surface on the entire primary dentition and permanent molars.

11   Natural movement of all the teeth over time toward the midline of the oral cavity.

12   Parafunctional habit of grinding the teeth.

15   First dentition present, also called the *deciduous dentition.*

16   Side to which the mandible has been moved during lateral occlusion.

17   Type of terminal plane or _____ relationship in which the primary mandibular second molar is mesial to the maxillary molar.

18   Space created when the primary molars are shed to make room for the much smaller mesiodistal permanent premolars.

20   Other side of the arch from the working side during lateral occlusion.

24   Facial profile that usually shows a rather prominent mandible and possibly a normal or even retrusive maxilla or concave profile.

26   End point of closure of the mandible in which the mandible is in the most retruded position is _____ relationship.

27   Lowering of the lower jaw.

28   Moving the lower jaw backward.

Down:

1   Failure to have an overall ideal form to the dentition while in centric occlusion.

2   Cusps that function during centric occlusion and include the lingual cusps of the maxillary posterior teeth and the buccal cusps of the mandibular posterior teeth, as well as the incisal edges of the mandibular anterior teeth.

4   Situation in which the maxillary dental arch overhangs the mandibular arch facially.

5   Spaces between certain primary teeth.

8   Situation in which the maxillary incisors also overlap the mandibular incisors.

13   Facial profile in centric occlusion with slightly protruded jaws, giving the facial outline a relatively flat appearance or straight profile.

14   If imaginary planes are placed on the masticatory surfaces of each dental arch, the maxillary arch is convex occlusally and the mandibular arch is concave, producing an anteroposterior curvature.

19   Concave curve results when a frontal section is taken through each set of both maxillary and mandibular molars, the firsts, seconds, and then thirds.

21   Parafunctional habit in which the teeth are held in centric occlusion for long periods without a break into interocclusal clearance.

22   Situation in which the canine should be the only tooth in function during lateral occlusion.

23   Bony projection off the posterior and superior border of the mandibular ramus.

25   Occusal _____ to the periodontium resulting from occlusal disharmony.

Words to Find

Anatomical	Cusp	Interproximal	Permanent
Axis	Deciduous	Masticatory	Primary
Cementoenamel	Dentition	Mesial	Proximal
Clinical	Distal	Midline	Quadrants
Concavities	Embrasures	Occlusal	Sextants
Contact	Incisal	Occlusion	Thirds
Contour	International	Palmer	Universal

Word Search, Puzzle 1

```
A I A J G I N T E R P R O X I M A L O Q
T H I R D S T L T L R V F L Y R V S B L
P K L N B C F N T M X U A L U C T H E L
N S O Z A A E G Y D A I O O T N A M B L
I F S T K N V W M C S S T C A C A X A J
C S N Z A A U E O E O N T T C N K N I L
T O V M B T N T M K O N X I E L O X A S
C C R P S O I G E C V E C O C I U M L C
H E U Q K M V S J N S O T A T A I S Y E
P N W S K I E D J Q D N C A V X T Q A L
L R L R P C R B U E E I N C O I N O A L
W V I E R A S Q K M M R S R L B T C R S
Z C N M D L A U E R E B P T C U I I U Y
B J C V A H L C C T M P R V A N S O E R
K M I F X R F K N P F C Y A I L U I E S
Q A S F U V Y I A I Z S V L S D U M O I
Z W A U X O N R J M S J C Q I U L E E N
O M L Q U A D R A N T S Z C F A R K D T
X W D E N T I T I O N D E K P Q Z E D D
O H M I D L I N E J H D T W N U Q X S P
```

Words to Find

Anodontia	Cuspids	Furcation	Peg
Avulsion	Dentigerous	Impacted	Supernumerary
Bicuspid	Diastema	Mamelons	Supplemental
Bifurcated	Dilaceration	Marginal	Transverse
Carabelli	Eminence	Mesiodens	Triangular
Central	Flutting	Mulberry	Trifurcated
Cingulum	Fossa	Multirooted	Tubercles

Word Search, Puzzle 2

```
P K A C B B I F U R C A T E D E U F F M
U O A I B T O S T Y E N L W D T D X R D
S I Z N N B I J U S W A U E D I O A E A
F M C G K A D M R P T S T D P Y L T A Q
L P J U T G K E A N E O N S Q U A S Y H
U A K L L Z V I E I O R U P G C S G E F
T C W U Y S T M G R S C N N R O R M F V
T T S M N N E L I L I K A U F O V F X E
I E U A O L H T L B H I F D M F X A R I
N D R D P W L Q D U R I Z I Z E X I Y Q
G T O P D U Y A E T R D X L Z I R G Q N
R N U R M F B T N T P C M A M S H A P P
A S M M E U K U T D E A A C P E A I R S
V C U A S R N B I I G R R E N M V C F Y
A U L M I C D E G A S A G R G I U E J L
P S B E O A H R E S L B I A O N L N X C
P P E L D T L C R T Z E N T D E S T D C
X I R O E I C L O E X L A I P N I R D O
I D R N N O B E U M K L L O S C O A D Y
U S Y S S N O S S A B I P N T E N L V X
```

Words to Find

Abfraction	Deviation	Overjet	Step
Articular	Disc	Parafunctional	Subluxation
Balancing	Drift	Premature	Supporting
Bruxism	Elevation	Primary	Synovial
Capsule	Group	Primate	Temporomandibular
Centric	Interocclusal	Prognathic	Terminal
Cervical	Leeway	Protrusion	Trauma
Clenching	Malocclusion	Retraction	Wilson
Condyle	Mesognathic	Retrognathic	Working
Crossbite	Occlusion	Rise	
Depression	Overbite	Spee	

Word Search, Puzzle 3

```
A  U  F  P  R  I  M  A  T  E  R  E  T  R  A  C  T  I  O  N
R  I  N  T  E  R  O  C  C  L  U  S  A  L  W  I  L  S  O  N
T  O  N  T  E  M  P  O  R  O  M  A  N  D  I  B  U  L  A  R
I  P  G  X  E  L  E  V  A  T  I  O  N  P  R  I  M  A  R  Y
C  O  N  D  Y  L  E  M  A  L  O  C  C  L  U  S  I  O  N  J
U  S  P  M  D  S  U  B  L  U  X  A  T  I  O  N  R  I  S  E
L  P  W  O  R  K  I  N  G  B  P  R  O  G  N  A  T  H  I  C
A  W  R  X  M  E  S  O  G  N  A  T  H  I  C  D  R  I  F  T
R  R  A  E  V  V  C  E  I  U  P  M  T  E  R  M  I  N  A  L
H  C  E  O  M  L  E  E  W  A  Y  D  E  V  I  A  T  I  O  N
D  L  P  T  M  A  P  A  R  A  F  U  N  C  T  I  O  N  A  L
E  E  B  R  R  X  T  T  O  V  E  R  B  I  T  E  S  T  E  P
P  N  A  S  O  O  Z  U  C  R  O  S  S  B  I  T  E  O  T  J
R  C  L  B  C  T  G  Q  R  T  F  O  C  C  L  U  S  I  O  N
E  H  A  R  T  E  R  N  C  E  R  V  I  C  A  L  S  P  E  E
S  I  N  U  R  G  N  U  A  V  A  B  F  R  A  C  T  I  O  N
S  N  C  X  A  R  D  T  S  T  S  U  P  P  O  R  T  I  N  G
I  G  I  I  U  O  I  X  R  I  H  H  S  Y  N  O  V  I  A  L
O  H  N  S  M  U  S  D  Y  I  O  I  X  O  V  E  R  J  E  T
N  W  G  M  A  P  C  Q  L  I  C  N  C  C  A  P  S  U  L  E
```

Guidelines
for Tooth
Drawing

Introduction

Tooth-drawing assignments emphasize fundamental principles in tooth design, which later have practical application in clinical course work. Initial drawings are most likely to be the student's first attempts at capturing toothlikenesses; they will certainly encourage accuracy and discernment of the teeth and hopefully facilitate the recognition of tooth details. Artistic inclinations are not really needed with these basic technical drawings.

It is important also to note that these drawings are two dimensional only and are somewhat limited to fundamental outlines and proportions. However, they will serve to help create mental pictures of teeth in their ideal or composite state. Remember also that real specimens in patients' mouths vary considerably.

Activity

1. Locate gridded worksheets in the workbook. Any additional gridded worksheets can be easily photocopied. Correctly label the worksheet at the top of the page with the tooth name and number that will be drawn.

2. Using attached table of tooth dimensions (same as in the textbook), mark off the overall peripheral tooth measurements for each of the gridded view boxes of the tooth. Note that the grid of the worksheet is larger than that shown with the tooth outlines to better enable the student to have room to work. Each square of grid equals one millimeter, so just count off as many squares for each peripheral dimension (such as the mesiodistal diameter) as indicated from the table onto the proper area of the gridded worksheet.

3. To establish crown and root proportions, divide each gridded view box, into two parts corresponding to these two dimensions except for the incisal/occlusal view.

4. To indicate the height of contour, locate the approximate area of contact between the adjacent teeth and the area of greatest convexity on the labial/buccal, lingual and mesial, and distal surfaces as mentioned in the textbook.

5. To locate the root axis line (RAL), draw a line which exactly bisects the overall gridded box showing the overall crown and root measurements. The CEJ will then be bisected by this RAL. The root apex may or may not be located on this RAL depending on the tooth' apex traits.

6. To locate the center of the cingulum or midpoint of the incisal edge, divide the crown and root (if included in that particular gridded view box) into imaginary thirds. Then place the root apex, cingulum or incisal edge into proper perspective with respect to the other peripheral overall tooth dimensions such as the mesio-distal diameter.

7. To complete the crown outline, connect the heights of contour to the incisal/occlusal edge, to the CEJ, as well as to the other heights of contour. Any additional anatomical features such as mamelons, lobes, marginal ridges, depressions, etc. can be indicated upon completion of the crown outline.

8. To complete the root outline, follow the directions for developing the crown outline with the understanding that the cervical one third to one half of the root width generally approximates the cervical width of the crown before it starts to narrow considerably to form the root apex.

9. Shading or stippling of the features may now be added if desired. An evaluation form for the drawings for use by both the student and instructor is also included in the workbook. Multiple copies of the form may be photocopied.

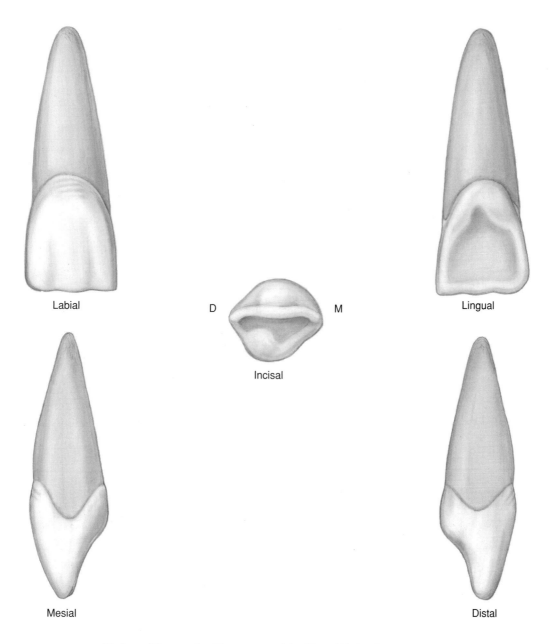

Labial

Lingual

D   M

Incisal

Mesial

Distal

Various Views of a Permanent Maxillary Right Central Incisor

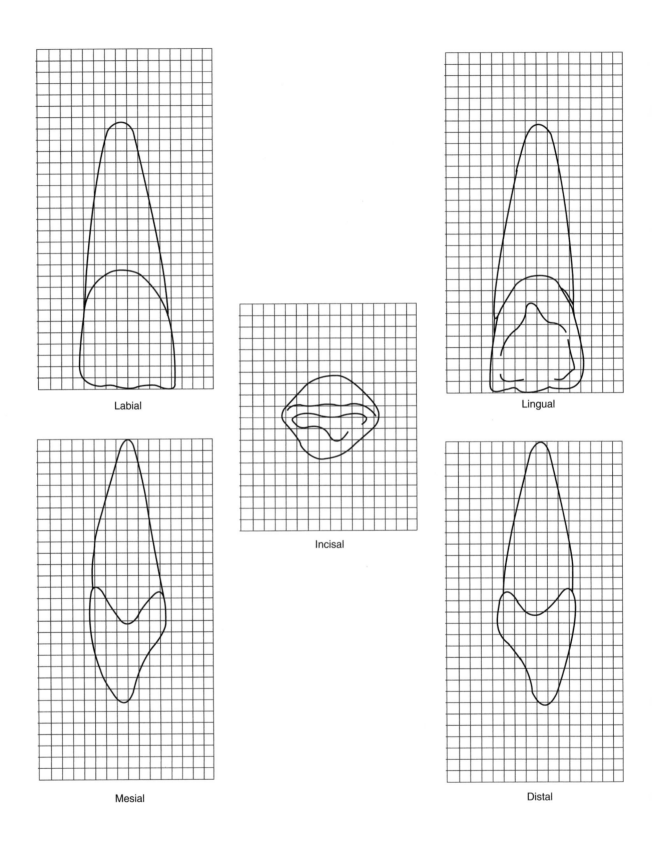

Labial

Lingual

Incisal

Mesial

Distal

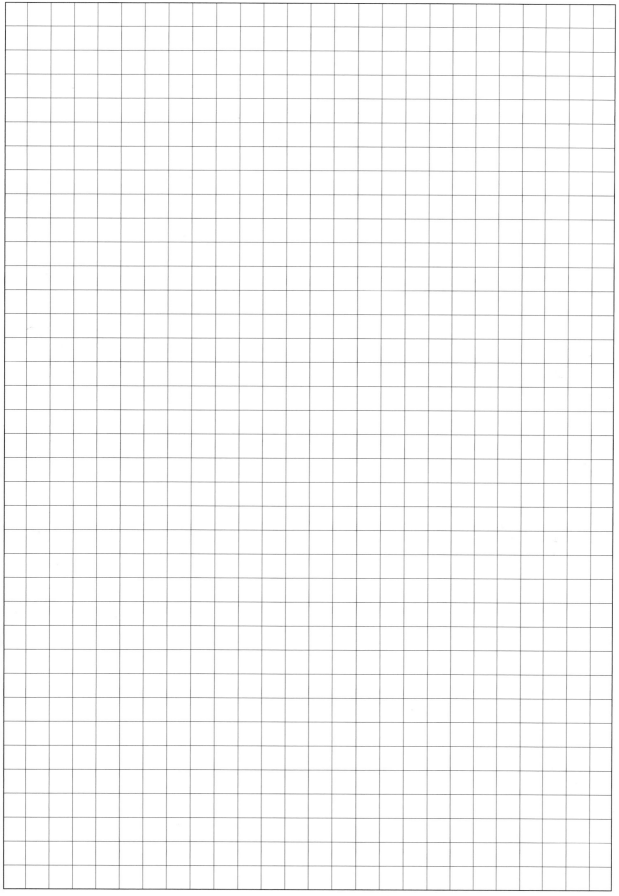

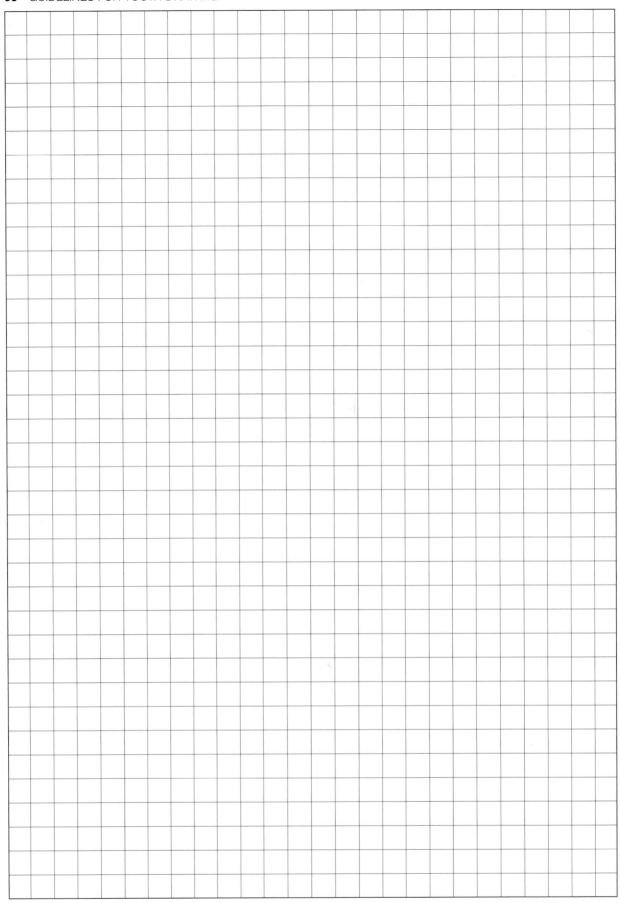

DIMENSIONS OF PERMANENT MAXILLARY CENTRAL INCISOR*

Cervicoincisal Length of Crown	10.5
Length of Root	13.0
Mesiodistal Diameter of Crown	8.5
Mesiodistal Diameter at CEJ	7.0
Labiolingual Diameter	7.0
Labiolingual Diameter at CEJ	6.0
Curvature of CEJ—Mesial	3.5
Curvature of CEJ—Distal	2.5

*Information adapted from Ash MM, Nelson *SJ: Wheeler's Dental Anatomy, Physiology and Occlusion*, ed 8, WB Saunders, Philadelphia, 2003.

CHECKLIST FOR PERMANENT MAXILLARY CENTRAL INCISOR

Features Noted	Features Present
Crown Features	
Incisal edge, mamelons, distal offset cingulum, wide and shallow lingual fossa, longer mesial than distal marginal ridges, and linguoincisal edge	
Sharper MI incisal angle, rounder DI angle, and more pronounced mesial CEJ curvature	
Height of contour in cervical third	
Mesial contact is just cervical to the junction of occlusal and middle thirds	
Distal contact is at junction of incisal and middle thirds	
Root Features	
Single rooted, overall conical shape, rounded apex	
No proximal root concavities	

Name _____   Tooth Number/Name _____

Date _____   Instructor Rating _____

DRAWING EVALUATION CHECKLIST

RATING SCALE

Fully Correct = 2 points   Major Error = 0 points

Minor Error = 1 point   Note: NA (non-appropriate)

SELF EVALUATION RATING

FIVE VIEWS	Clearly Drawn	Accurate Sizing	General Features Included	Specific Features Included
1. Facial View				
2. Lingual View				
3. Mesial View				
4. Distal View				
5. Incisal/ Occlusal View				

Self Evaluation Rating = $\dfrac{\text{points received}}{\text{points possible}}$ = _____ = _____ %

INSTRUCTOR EVALUATION RATING

FIVE VIEWS	Clearly Drawn	Accurate Sizing	General Features Included	Specific Features Included
1. Facial View				
2. Lingual View				
3. Mesial View				
4. Distal View				
5. Incisal/ Occlusal View				

Instructor Evaluation Rating = $\dfrac{\text{points received}}{\text{points possible}}$ = _____ = _____ %

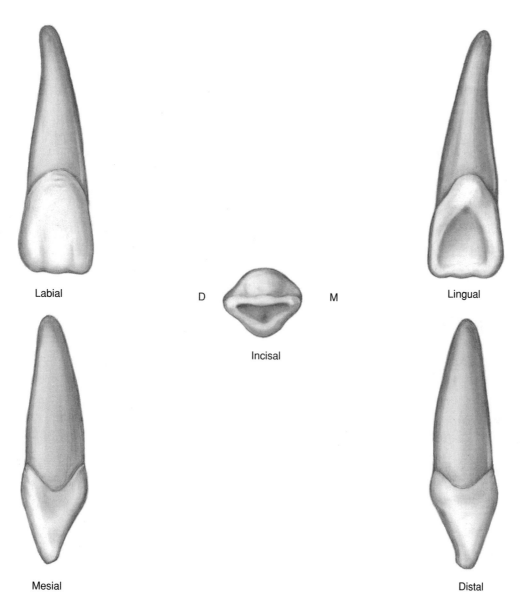

Labial

D

M

Lingual

Incisal

Mesial

Distal

Various Views of a Permanent Maxillary Right Lateral Incisor

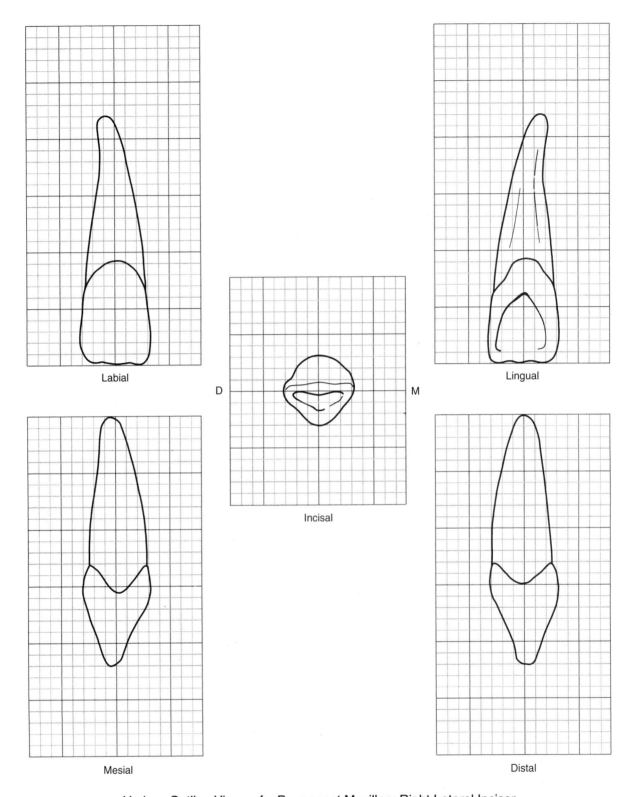

Labial

Lingual

D   M

Incisal

Mesial

Distal

Various Outline Views of a Permanent Maxillary Right Lateral Incisor

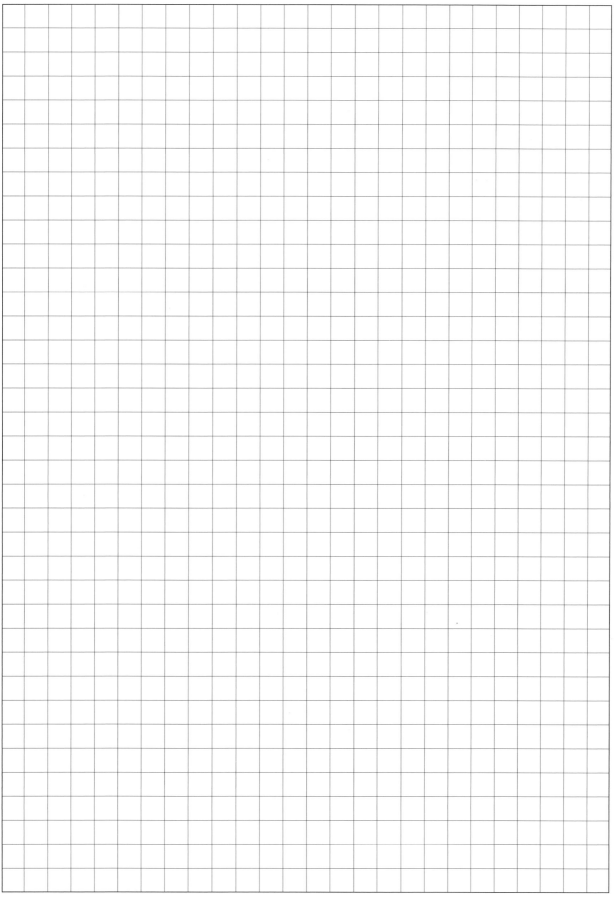

DIMENSIONS OF PERMANENT MAXILLARY LATERAL INCISOR*	
Cervico-incisal Length of Crown	9.0
Length of Root	13.0
Mesiodistal Diameter of Crown	6.5
Mesiodistal Diameter at CEJ	5.0
Labiolingual Diameter	6.0
Labiolingual Diameter at CEJ	5.0
Curvature of CEJ—Mesial	3.0
Curvature of CEJ—Distal	2.0

* Information adapted from Ash MM, Nelson SJ: *Wheeler's Dental Anatomy, Physiology and Occlusion*, ed 8, WB Saunders, Philadelphia, 2003.

CHECKLIST FOR PERMANENT MAXILLARY LATERAL INCISOR	
Features Noted	**Features Present**
Crown Features	
Incisal edge, mamelons, centered and narrow cingulum, deep lingual fossa, pronounced marginal ridges, and linguoincisal ridge	
Sharper MI incisal angle, rounder DI angle, and more pronounced mesial CEJ curvature	
Height of contour in cervical third	
Mesial contact is just cervical to the junction of occlusal and middle thirds	
Distal contact is at middle third or junction with incisal third	
Root Features	
Single rooted, overall conical shape, root curve to the distal, with sharp apex	
No proximal root concavities and the same or longer than central, yet thinner	

Name _____   Tooth Number/Name _____

Date _____   Instructor Rating _____

DRAWING EVALUATION CHECKLIST

RATING SCALE

Fully Correct = 2 points   Major Error = 0 points
Minor Error = 1 point   Note: NA (non-appropriate)

SELF EVALUATION RATING

FIVE VIEWS	Clearly Drawn	Accurate Sizing	General Features Included	Specific Features Included
1. Facial View				
2. Lingual View				
3. Mesial View				
4. Distal View				
5. Incisal/ Occlusal View				

Self Evaluation Rating = $\dfrac{\text{points received}}{\text{points possible}}$ = _____ = _____ %

INSTRUCTOR EVALUATION RATING

FIVE VIEWS	Clearly Drawn	Accurate Sizing	General Features Included	Specific Features Included
1. Facial View				
2. Lingual View				
3. Mesial View				
4. Distal View				
5. Incisal/ Occlusal View				

Instructor Evaluation Rating = $\dfrac{\text{points received}}{\text{points possible}}$ = _____ = _____ %

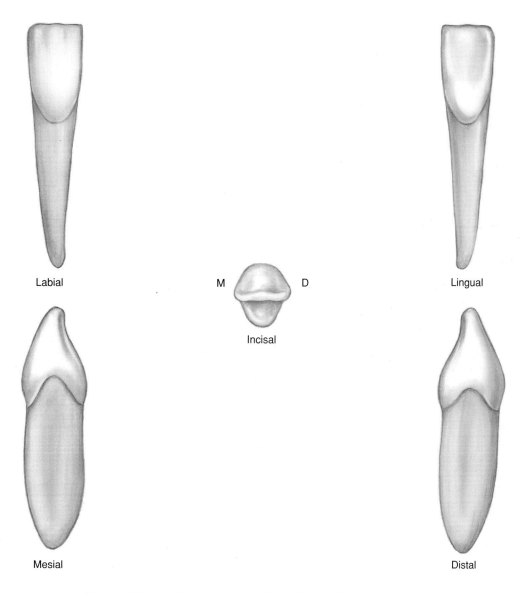

Labial

M   D

Incisal

Lingual

Mesial

Distal

Various Views of a Permanent Mandibular Right Central Incisor

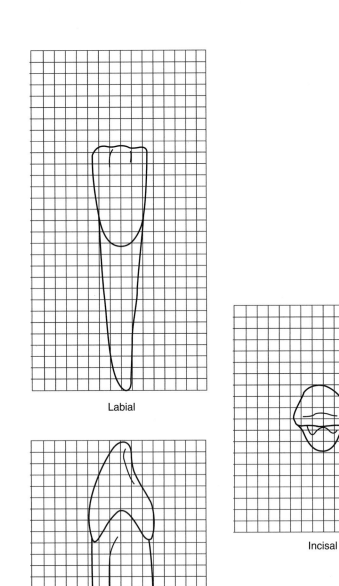

Labial

Incisal

Mesial

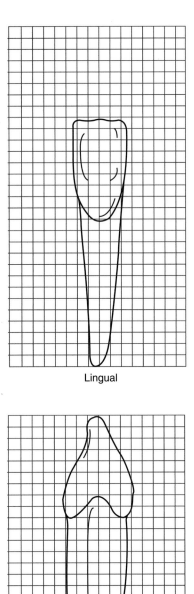

Lingual

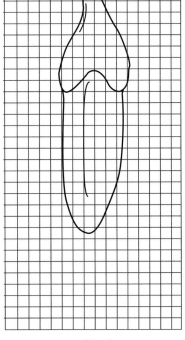

Distal

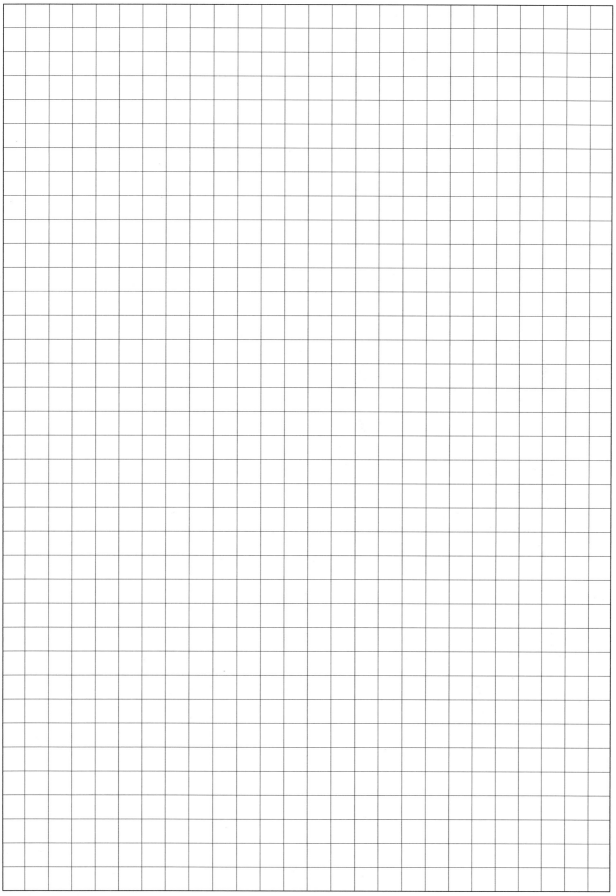

DIMENSIONS OF PERMANENT MANDIBULAR CENTRAL INCISOR*

Cervico-incisal Length of Crown	Buccal: 9.0 Lingual: 9.5
Length of Root	12.5
Mesiodistal Diameter of Crown	5.0
Mesiodistal Diameter at CEJ	3.5
Labiolingual Diameter	6.0
Labiolingual Diameter at CEJ	5.3
Curvature of CEJ—Mesial	3.0
Curvature of CEJ—Distal	2.0

* Information adapted from Ash MM, Nelson SJ: *Wheeler's Dental Anatomy, Physiology and Occlusion*, ed 8, WB Saunders, Philadelphia, 2003.

CHECKLIST FOR PERMANENT MANDIBULAR CENTRAL INCISOR

Features Noted	Features Present
Crown Features	
Bilaterally symmetrical	
Incisal edge, mamelons, small centered cingulum, subtle lingual fossa, and equal subtle marginal ridges	
Sharper MI incisal angle, rounder DI angle, and more pronounced mesial CEJ curvature	
Height of contour in cervical third	
Mesial contact is just cervical to the junction of occlusal and middle thirds	
Distal contact is at incisal third	
Root Features	
Single rooted, with root longer than the crown	
Proximal root concavities give double-rooted appearance	

Name _____   Tooth Number/Name _____

Date _____   Instructor Rating _____

DRAWING EVALUATION CHECKLIST

RATING SCALE

Fully Correct = 2 points   Major Error = 0 points
Minor Error = 1 point   Note: NA (non-appropriate)

SELF EVALUATION RATING

FIVE VIEWS	Clearly Drawn	Accurate Sizing	General Features Included	Specific Features Included
1. Facial View				
2. Lingual View				
3. Mesial View				
4. Distal View				
5. Incisal/ Occlusal View				

Self Evaluation Rating = $\dfrac{\text{points received}}{\text{points possible}}$ = _____ = _____ %

INSTRUCTOR EVALUATION RATING

FIVE VIEWS	Clearly Drawn	Accurate Sizing	General Features Included	Specific Features Included
1. Facial View				
2. Lingual View				
3. Mesial View				
4. Distal View				
5. Incisal/ Occlusal View				

Instructor Evaluation Rating = $\dfrac{\text{points received}}{\text{points possible}}$ = _____ = _____ %

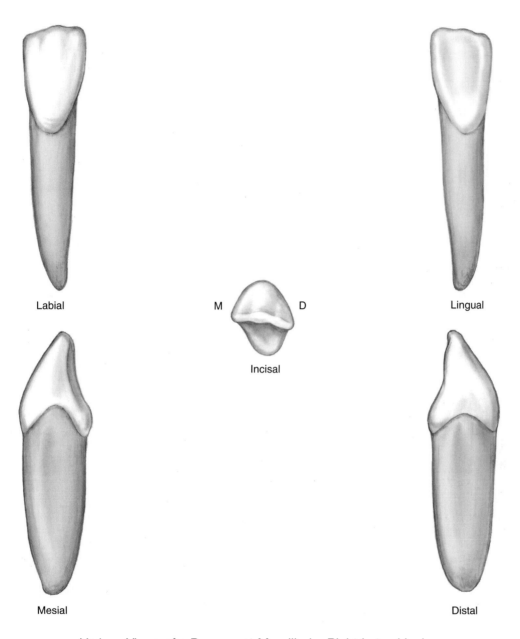

Labial

Lingual

M   D

Incisal

Mesial

Distal

Various Views of a Permanent Mandibular Right Lateral Incisor

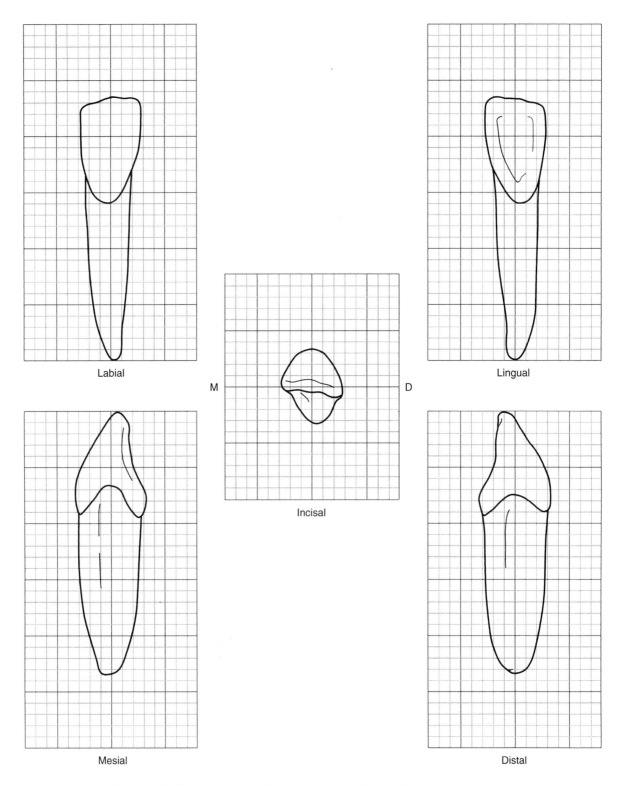

Labial

Lingual

M

D

Incisal

Mesial

Distal

Various Outline Views of a Permanent Mandibular Right Lateral Incisor

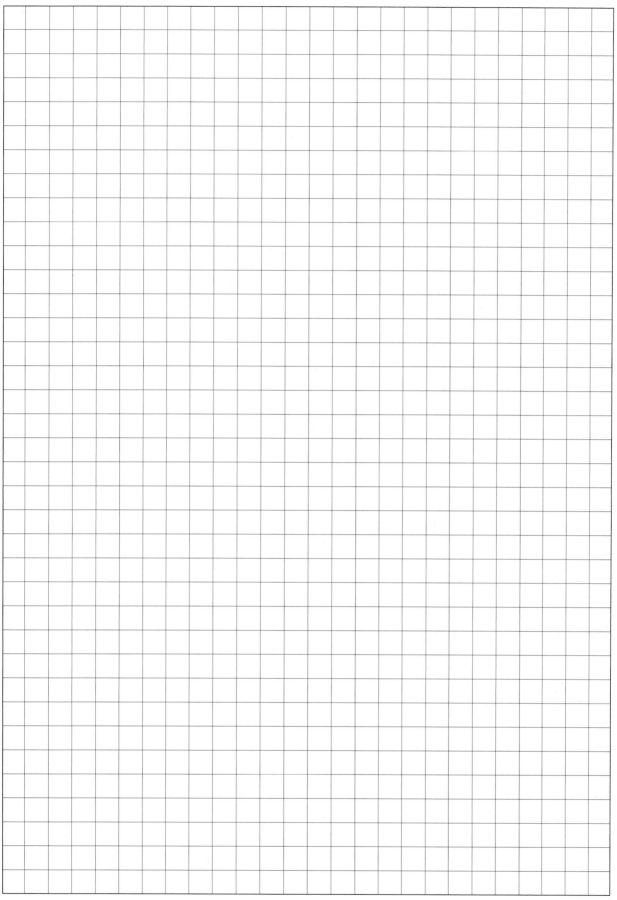

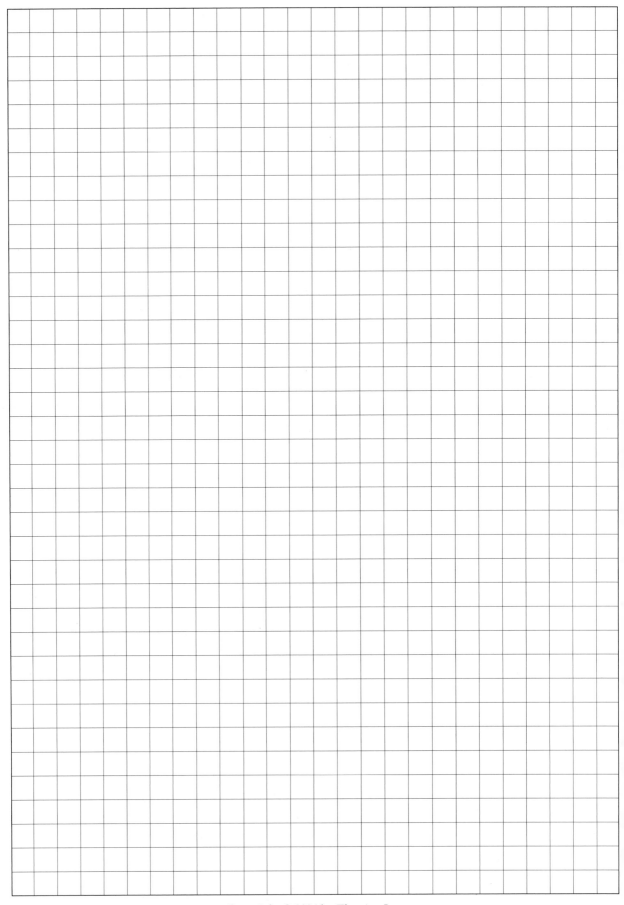

DIMENSIONS OF PERMANENT MANDIBULAR LATERAL INCISOR*

Cervico-incisal Length of Crown	Buccal: 9.5　　　Lingual: 10.0
Length of Root	14.0
Mesiodistal Diameter of Crown	5.5
Mesiodistal Diameter at CEJ	4.0
Labiolingual Diameter	6.5
Labiolingual Diameter at CEJ	5.8
Curvature of CEJ—Mesial	3.0
Curvature of CEJ—Distal	2.0

* Information adapted from Ash MM, Nelson SJ: *Wheeler's Dental Anatomy, Physiology and Occlusion,* ed 8, WB Saunders, Philadelphia, 2003.

CHECKLIST FOR PERMANENT MANDIBULAR LATERAL INCISOR

Features Noted	Features Present
Crown Features	
Larger than central and not bilaterally symmetrical, and appears twisted distally	
Incisal edge, mamelons, small distally displaced cingulum, lingual fossa, and moderate mesial marginal ridge longer than distal	
Sharper MI incisal angle, rounder DI angle, and more pronounced mesial CEJ curvature	
Height of contour in cervical third	
Mesial contact is just cervical to the junction of occlusal and middle thirds	
Distal contact is at incisal third	
Root Features	
Single rooted, with root longer than the crown	
Proximal root concavities give double-rooted appearance	

Name _____   Tooth Number/Name _____

Date _____   Instructor Rating _____

DRAWING EVALUATION CHECKLIST

RATING SCALE
Fully Correct = 2 points   Major Error = 0 points
Minor Error = 1 point   Note: NA (non-appropriate)

SELF EVALUATION RATING

FIVE VIEWS	Clearly Drawn	Accurate Sizing	General Features Included	Specific Features Included
1. Facial View				
2. Lingual View				
3. Mesial View				
4. Distal View				
5. Incisal/ Occlusal View				

Self Evaluation Rating = $\dfrac{\text{points received}}{\text{points possible}}$ = _____ = _____ %

INSTRUCTOR EVALUATION RATING

FIVE VIEWS	Clearly Drawn	Accurate Sizing	General Features Included	Specific Features Included
1. Facial View				
2. Lingual View				
3. Mesial View				
4. Distal View				
5. Incisal/ Occlusal View				

Instructor Evaluation Rating = $\dfrac{\text{points received}}{\text{points possible}}$ = _____ = _____ %

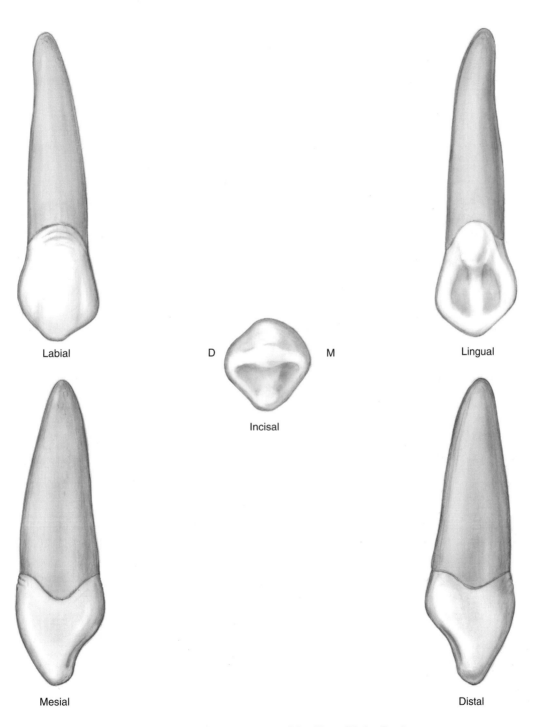

Labial

D   M

Incisal

Lingual

Mesial

Distal

Various Views of a Permanent Maxillary Right Canine

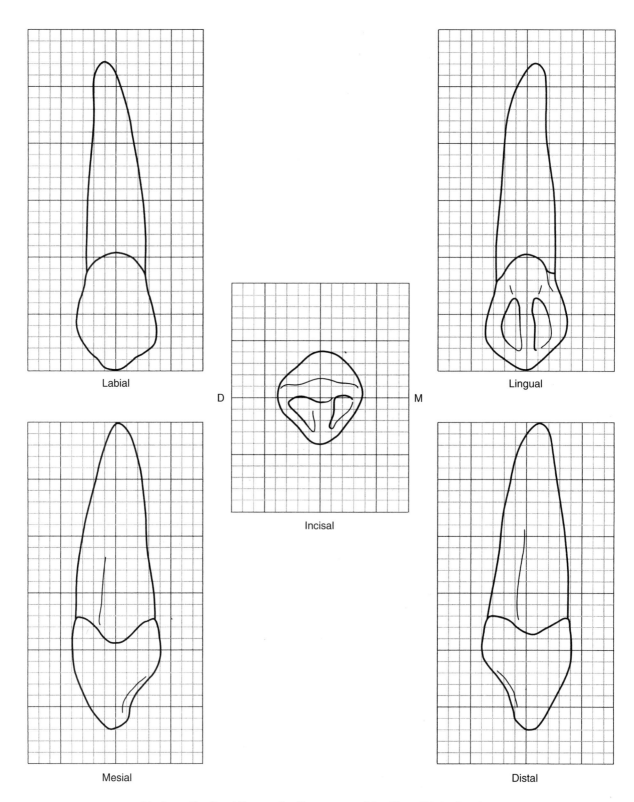

Labial

Incisal

Lingual

D M

Mesial

Distal

Various Outline Views of a Permanent Maxillary Right Canine

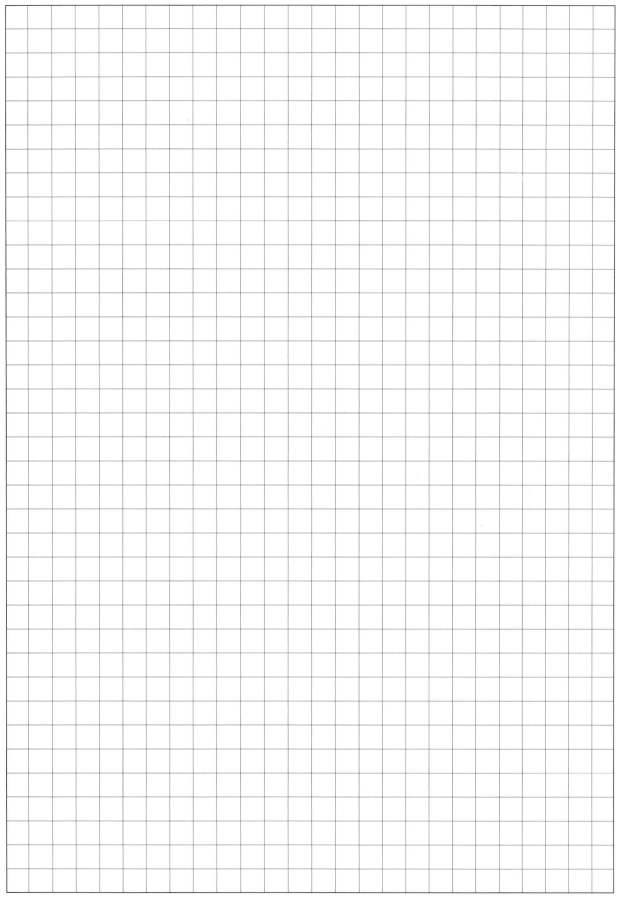

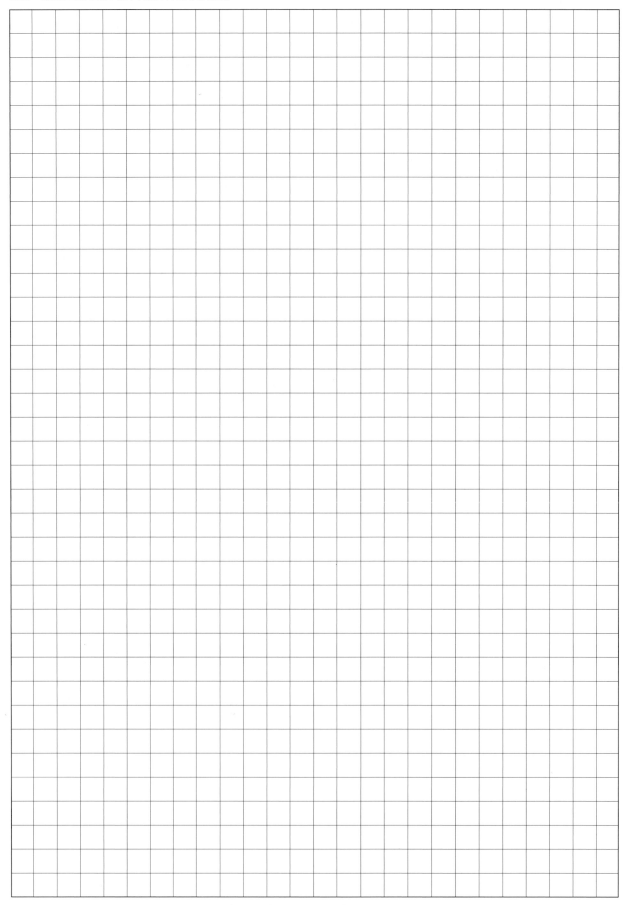

DIMENSIONS OF PERMANENT MAXILLARY CANINE*	
Cervico-incisal Length of Crown	10.0
Length of Root	17.0
Mesiodistal Diameter of Crown	7.5
Mesiodistal Diameter at CEJ	5.5
Labiolingual Diameter	8.0
Labiolingual Diameter at CEJ	7.0
Curvature of CEJ—Mesial	2.5
Curvature of CEJ—Distal	1.5

* Information adapted from Ash MM, Nelson SJ: *Wheeler's Dental Anatomy, Physiology and Occlusion*, ed 8, WB Saunders, Philadelphia, 2003.

CHECKLIST FOR PERMANENT MAXILLARY CANINE	
Features Noted	**Features Present**
Crown Features	
Single cusp, with sharp cusp tip and slopes, labial ridge	
Shorter mesial cusp slope, more cervical contact on distal, more pronounced mesial CEJ curvature	
Shorter distal outline on labial view with depression between the distal contact and CEJ	
Prominent lingual anatomy with marginal ridges and lingual ridge, cingulum, and lingual fossae	
Height of contour for buccal is cervical third and for lingual is middle third	
Mesial contact is at junction of incisal third and middle thirds	
Distal contact is at middle third	
Root Features	
Long, thick single root with proximal root concavities	
Blunt root apex	

Name _____   Tooth Number/Name _____

Date _____   Instructor Rating _____

DRAWING EVALUATION CHECKLIST

RATING SCALE

Fully Correct = 2 points   Major Error = 0 points
Minor Error = 1 point   Note: NA (non-appropriate)

SELF EVALUATION RATING

FIVE VIEWS	Clearly Drawn	Accurate Sizing	General Features Included	Specific Features Included
1. Facial View				
2. Lingual View				
3. Mesial View				
4. Distal View				
5. Incisal/ Occlusal View				

Self Evaluation Rating = $\dfrac{\text{points received}}{\text{points possible}}$ = _____ = _____ %

INSTRUCTOR EVALUATION RATING

FIVE VIEWS	Clearly Drawn	Accurate Sizing	General Features Included	Specific Features Included
1. Facial View				
2. Lingual View				
3. Mesial View				
4. Distal View				
5. Incisal/ Occlusal View				

Instructor Evaluation Rating = $\dfrac{\text{points received}}{\text{points possible}}$ = _____ = _____ %

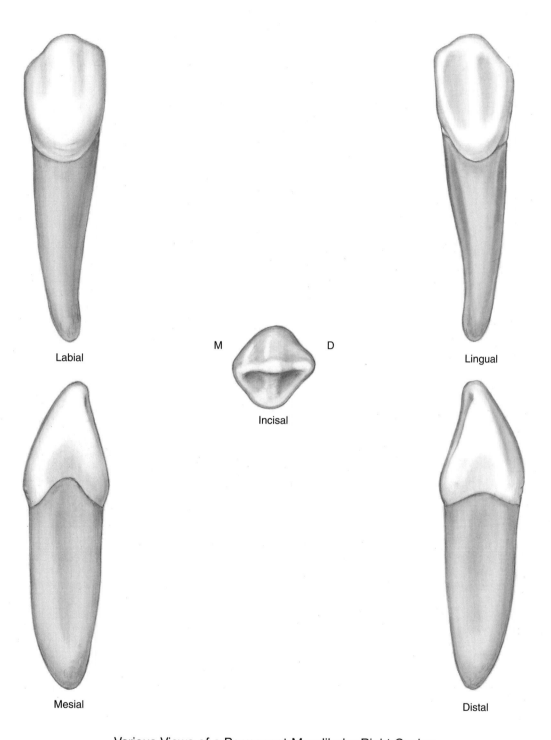

Labial

Lingual

M   D

Incisal

Mesial

Distal

Various Views of a Permanent Mandibular Right Canine

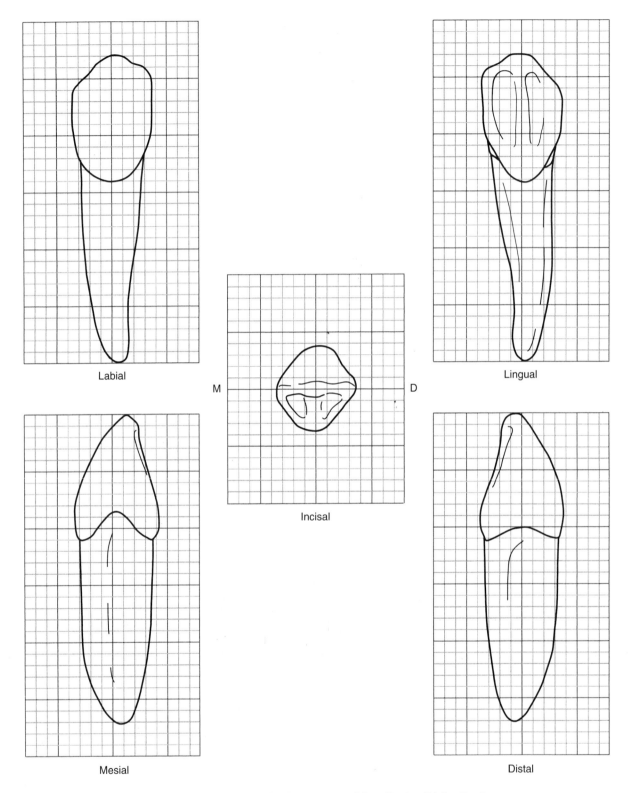

Labial

M

D

Incisal

Lingual

Mesial

Distal

Various Outline Views of a Permanent Mandibular Right Canine

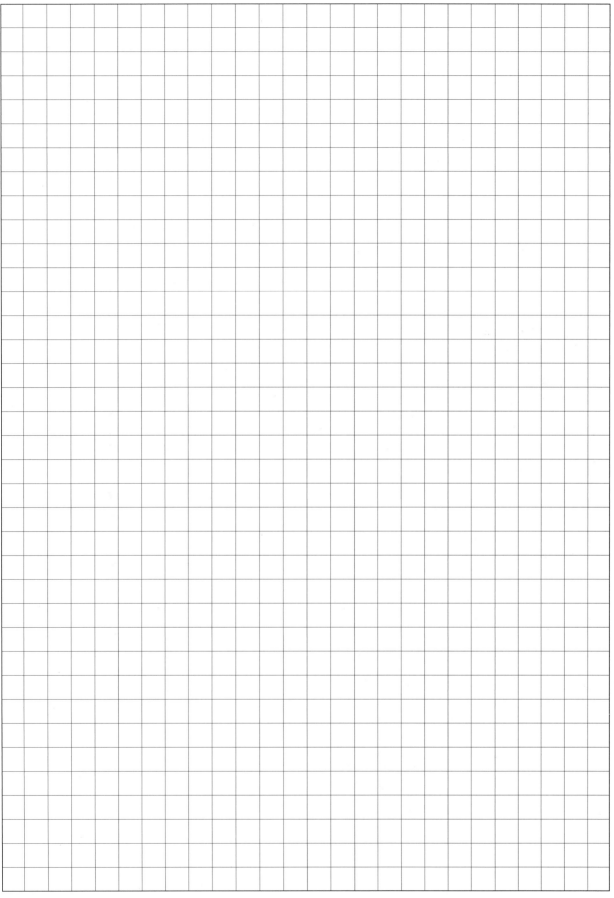

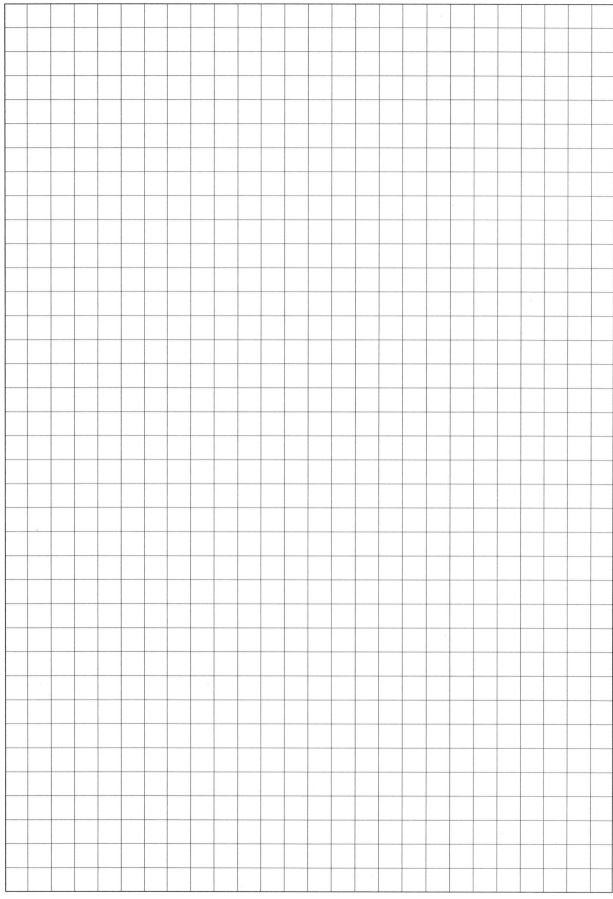

DIMENSIONS OF PERMANENT MANDIBULAR CANINE*	
Cervico-incisal Length of Crown	11.0
Length of Root	16.0
Mesiodistal Diameter of Crown	7.0
Mesiodistal Diameter at CEJ	5.5
Labiolingual Diameter	7.5
Labiolingual Diameter at CEJ	7
Curvature of CEJ—Mesial	2.5
Curvature of CEJ—Distal	1.0

*Information adapted from Ash MM, Nelson SJ: *Wheeler's Dental Anatomy, Physiology and Occlusion,* ed 8, WB Saunders, Philadelphia, 2003.

CHECKLIST FOR PERMANENT MANDIBULAR CANINE	
Features Noted	**Features Present**
Crown Features	
Single cusp, with less sharp cusp tip and slopes, labial ridge	
Shorter mesial cusp slope, more cervical contact on distal, more pronounced mesial CEJ curvature	
Shorter and rounder distal outline on labial view, with a shorter mesial slope than distal	
Smoother lingual anatomy	
Height of contour for buccal is cervical third and for lingual is middle third	
Mesial contact is at incisal thirds	
Distal contact is at junction of incisal and middle thirds	
Root Features	
Long, thick single root with proximal root concavities and with pointed apex	
Developmental depressions on mesial and distal give tooth double-rooted appearance	

Name _____   Tooth Number/Name _____

Date _____   Instructor Rating _____

DRAWING EVALUATION CHECKLIST

RATING SCALE

Fully Correct = 2 points   Major Error = 0 points
Minor Error = 1 point   Note: NA (non-appropriate)

SELF EVALUATION RATING

FIVE VIEWS	Clearly Drawn	Accurate Sizing	General Features Included	Specific Features Included
1. Facial View				
2. Lingual View				
3. Mesial View				
4. Distal View				
5. Incisal/ Occlusal View				

Self Evaluation Rating = $\dfrac{\text{points received}}{\text{points possible}}$ = _____ = _____ %

INSTRUCTOR EVALUATION RATING

FIVE VIEWS	Clearly Drawn	Accurate Sizing	General Features Included	Specific Features Included
1. Facial View				
2. Lingual View				
3. Mesial View				
4. Distal View				
5. Incisal/ Occlusal View				

Instructor Evaluation Rating = $\dfrac{\text{points received}}{\text{points possible}}$ = _____ = _____ %

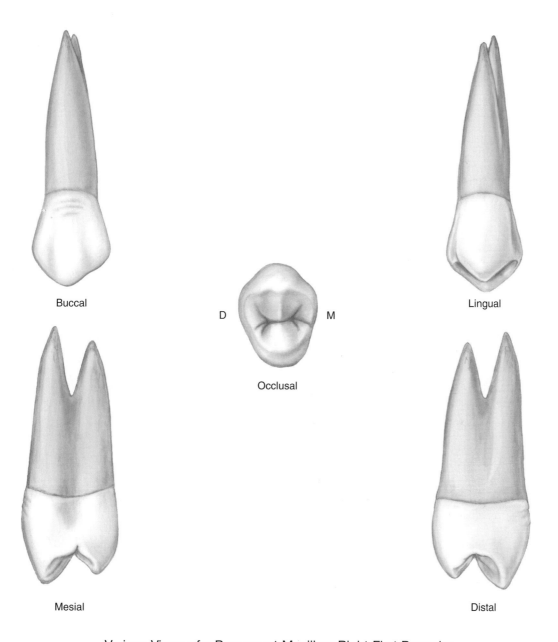

Buccal

D   M

Occlusal

Lingual

Mesial

Distal

Various Views of a Permanent Maxillary Right First Premolar

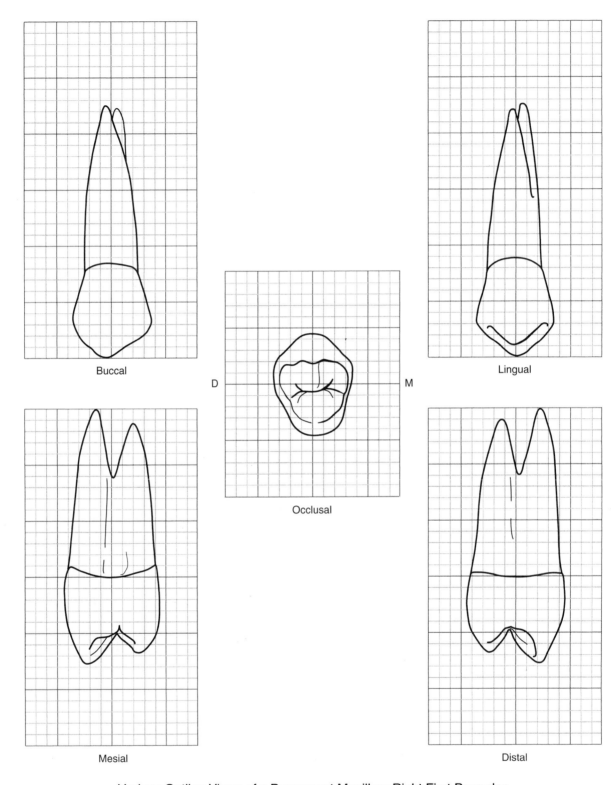

Buccal

Lingual

D   M

Occlusal

Mesial

Distal

Various Outline Views of a Permanent Maxillary Right First Premolar

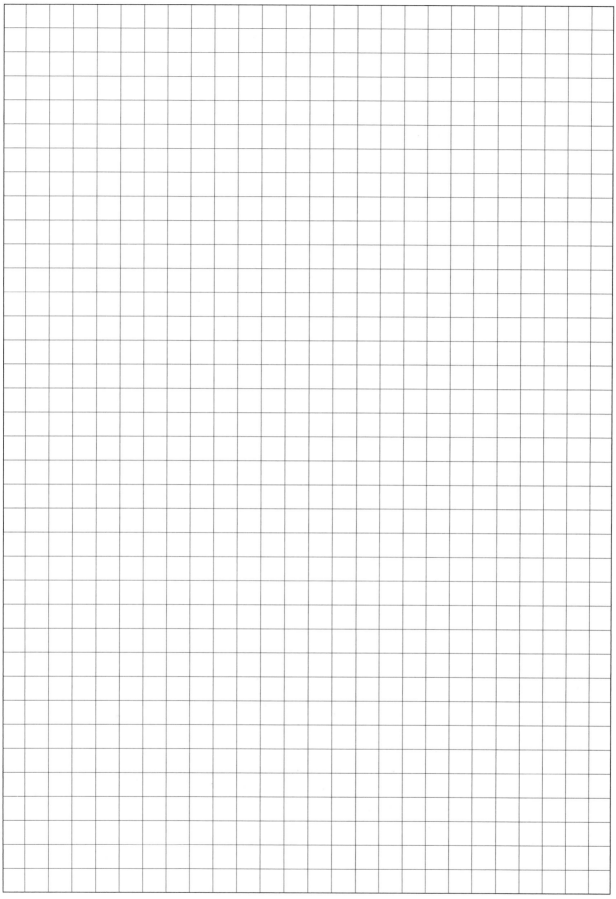

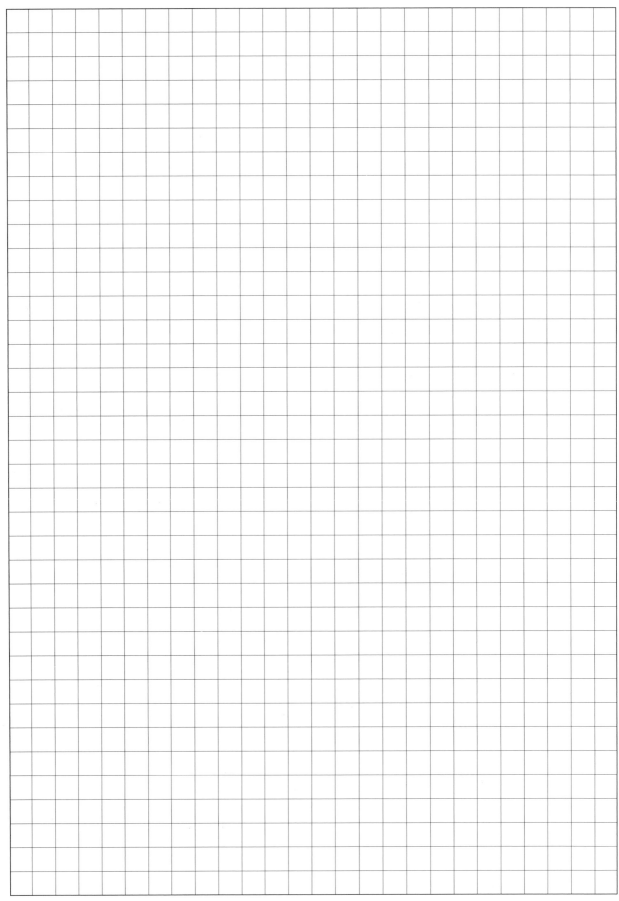

DIMENSIONS OF PERMANENT MAXILLARY FIRST PREMOLAR*	
Cervico-incisal Length of Crown	8.5
Length of Root	14.0
Mesiodistal Diameter of Crown	7.0
Mesiodistal Diameter at CEJ	5.0
Buccolingual Diameter	9.0
Buccolingual Diameter at CEJ	8.0
Curvature of CEJ—Mesial	1.0
Curvature of CEJ—Distal	0.0

*Information adapted from Ash MM, Nelson SJ: *Wheeler's Dental Anatomy, Physiology and Occlusion*, ed 8, WB Saunders, Philadelphia, 2003.

CHECKLIST FOR PERMANENT MAXILLARY FIRST PREMOLAR	
Features Noted	**Features Present**
Crown Features	
Buccal cusp longer of two with buccal ridge	
Occlusal table with marginal ridges and cusps, with tips, ridges, inclined planes, and grooves (long central groove), fossae, pits	
Longer mesial cusp slope, mesial marginal groove, mesial developmental depression, deeper mesial CEJ curvature	
Mesial and distal contact is just cervical to the junction of occlusal and middle thirds	
Root Features	
Bifurcated with root trunk	
Proximal root concavities	

Name _____   Tooth Number/Name _____

Date _____   Instructor Rating _____

DRAWING EVALUATION CHECKLIST

RATING SCALE

Fully Correct = 2 points   Major Error = 0 points
Minor Error = 1 point   Note: NA (non-appropriate)

SELF EVALUATION RATING

FIVE VIEWS	Clearly Drawn	Accurate Sizing	General Features Included	Specific Features Included
1. Facial View				
2. Lingual View				
3. Mesial View				
4. Distal View				
5. Incisal/ Occlusal View				

$$\text{Self Evaluation Rating} = \frac{\text{points received}}{\text{points possible}} = \underline{\hspace{2cm}} = \underline{\hspace{2cm}} \%$$

INSTRUCTOR EVALUATION RATING

FIVE VIEWS	Clearly Drawn	Accurate Sizing	General Features Included	Specific Features Included
1. Facial View				
2. Lingual View				
3. Mesial View				
4. Distal View				
5. Incisal/ Occlusal View				

$$\text{Instructor Evaluation Rating} = \frac{\text{points received}}{\text{points possible}} = \underline{\hspace{2cm}} = \underline{\hspace{2cm}} \%$$

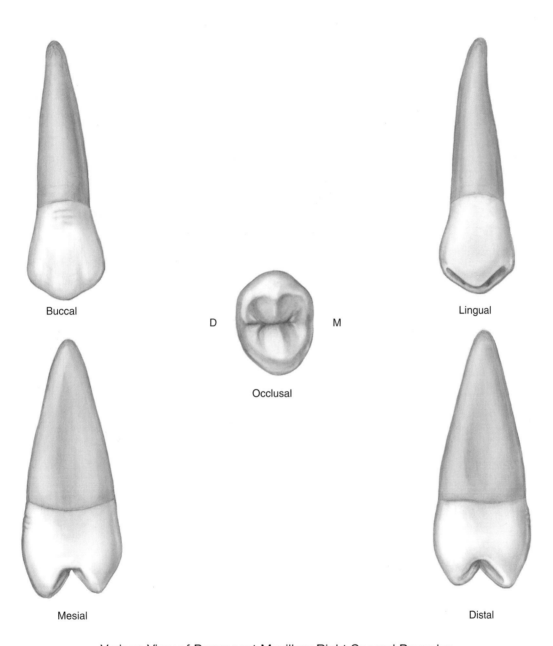

Buccal

D   M

Occlusal

Lingual

Mesial

Distal

Various View of Permanent Maxillary Right Second Premolar

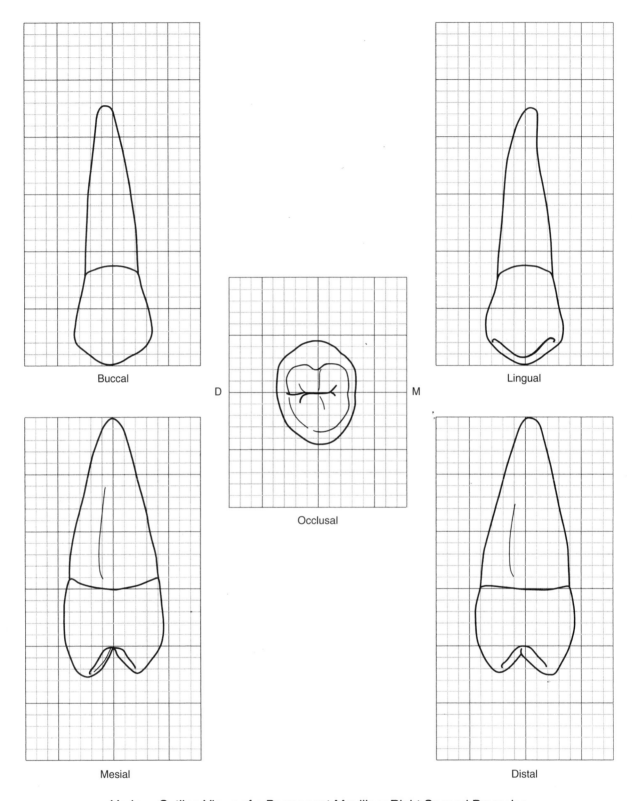

Buccal

D   Occlusal   M

Lingual

Mesial

Distal

Various Outline Views of a Permanent Maxillary Right Second Premolar

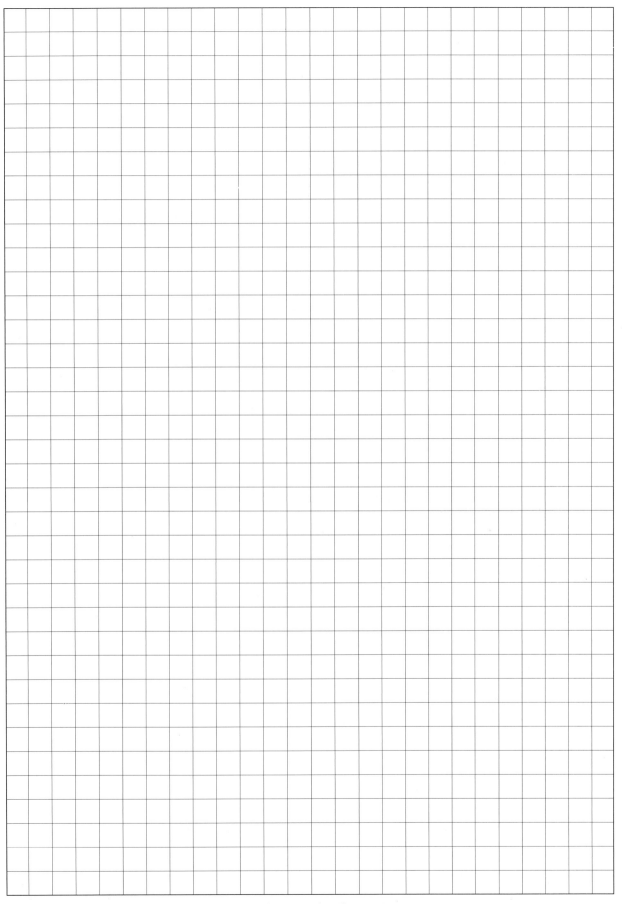

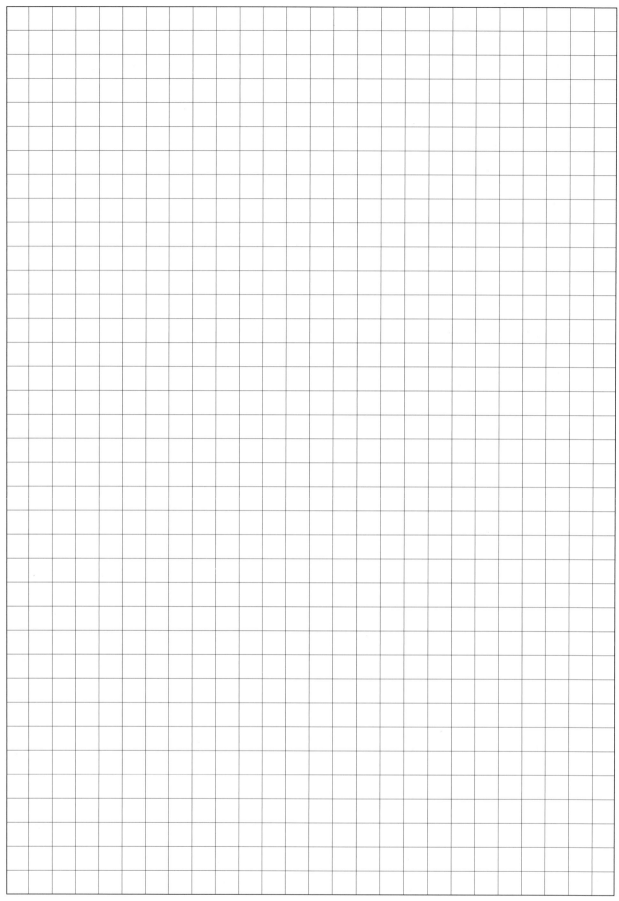

DIMENSIONS OF PERMANENT MAXILLARY SECOND PREMOLAR*	
Cervico-incisal Length of Crown	8.5
Length of Root	14.0
Mesiodistal Diameter of Crown	7.0
Mesiodistal Diameter at CEJ	5.0
Buccolingual Diameter	9.0
Buccolingual Diameter at CEJ	8.0
Curvature of CEJ—Mesial	1.0
Curvature of CEJ—Distal	0.0

*Information adapted from Ash MM, Nelson SJ: *Wheeler's Dental Anatomy, Physiology and Occlusion,* ed 8, WB Saunders, Philadelphia, 2003.

CHECKLIST FOR PERMANENT MAXILLARY SECOND PREMOLAR	
Features Noted	**Features Present**
Crown Features	
Two cusps same length with buccal ridge	
Occlusal table with marginal ridges and cusps, with tips, ridges, inclined planes, and grooves (short central groove and increased supplemental grooves), fossae, pits	
Lingual cusp offset to the mesial	
Mesial and distal contact is just cervical to the junction of occlusal and middle thirds	
Root Features	
Single rooted	
Proximal root concavities	

Name _____   Tooth Number/Name _____

Date _____   Instructor Rating _____

DRAWING EVALUATION CHECKLIST

RATING SCALE
Fully Correct = 2 points   Major Error = 0 points
Minor Error = 1 point   Note: NA (non-appropriate)

SELF EVALUATION RATING

FIVE VIEWS	Clearly Drawn	Accurate Sizing	General Features Included	Specific Features Included
1. Facial View				
2. Lingual View				
3. Mesial View				
4. Distal View				
5. Incisal/ Occlusal View				

Self Evaluation Rating = $\dfrac{\text{points received}}{\text{points possible}}$ = _____ = _____ %

INSTRUCTOR EVALUATION RATING

FIVE VIEWS	Clearly Drawn	Accurate Sizing	General Features Included	Specific Features Included
1. Facial View				
2. Lingual View				
3. Mesial View				
4. Distal View				
5. Incisal/ Occlusal View				

Instructor Evaluation Rating = $\dfrac{\text{points received}}{\text{points possible}}$ = _____ = _____ %

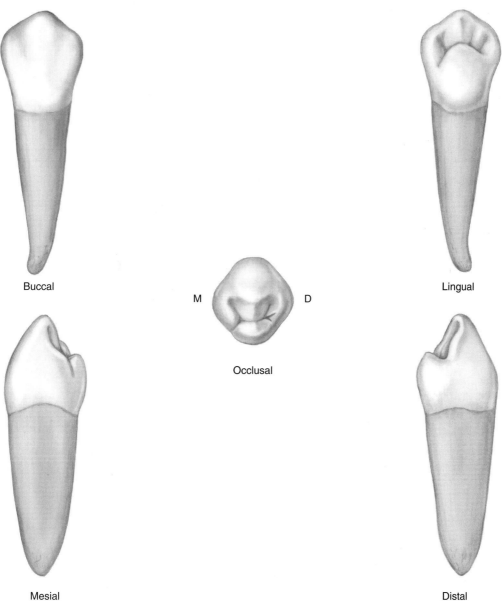

Buccal

Lingual

M   D

Occlusal

Mesial

Distal

Various Views of a Permanent Mandibular Right First Premolar

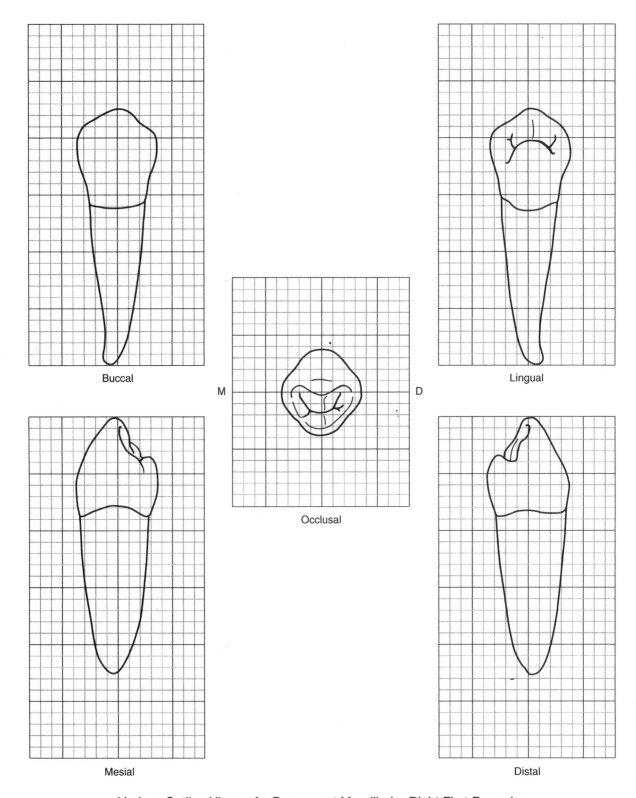

Buccal

Lingual

M   D

Occlusal

Mesial

Distal

Various Outline Views of a Permanent Mandibular Right First Premolar

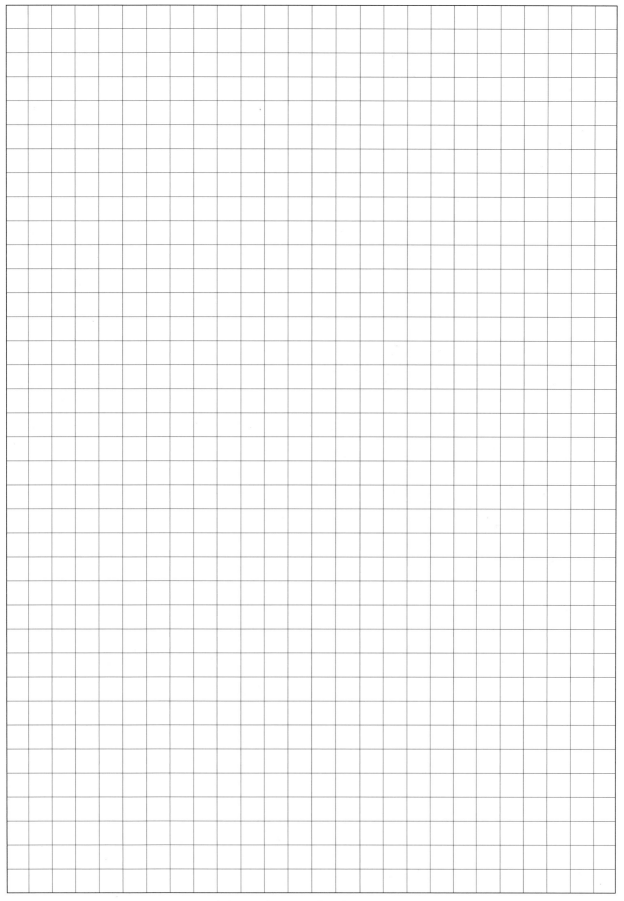

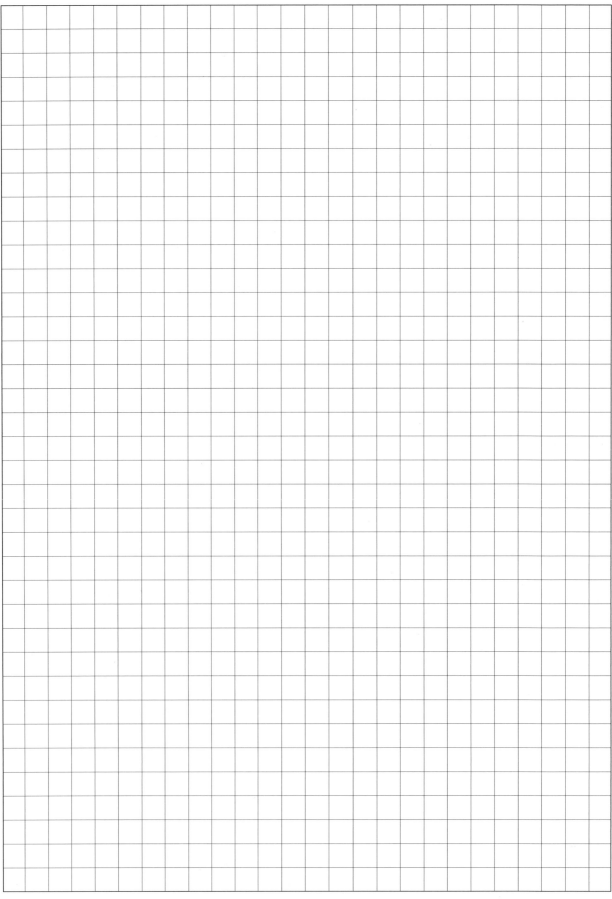

DIMENSIONS OF PERMANENT MANDIBULAR FIRST PREMOLAR*

Cervico-incisal Length of Crown	8.5
Length of Root	14.0
Mesiodistal Diameter of Crown	7.0
Mesiodistal Diameter at CEJ	5.0
Buccolingual Diameter	7.5
Buccolingual Diameter at CEJ	6.5
Curvature of CEJ—Mesial	1.0
Curvature of CEJ—Distal	0.0

*Information adapted from Ash MM: *Wheeler's Dental Anatomy, Physiology and Occlusion*, ed 8, WB Saunders, Philadelphia, 2002.

CHECKLIST FOR PERMANENT MANDIBULAR FIRST PREMOLAR

Features Noted	Features Present
Crown Features	
Smaller lingual cusp of two with buccal ridge	
Occlusal table with marginal ridges and cusps, with tips, ridges, inclined planes, and grooves, fossae, pits	
Shorter mesial cusp slope, mesiolingual groove, deeper mesial CEJ curvature	
Mesial and distal contact is just cervical to the junction of occlusal and middle thirds	
Root Features	
Single rooted	
Proximal root concavities	

Name _____   Tooth Number/Name _____

Date _____   Instructor Rating _____

DRAWING EVALUATION CHECKLIST

RATING SCALE

Fully Correct = 2 points   Major Error = 0 points
Minor Error = 1 point   Note: NA (non-appropriate)

SELF EVALUATION RATING

FIVE VIEWS	Clearly Drawn	Accurate Sizing	General Features Included	Specific Features Included
1. Facial View				
2. Lingual View				
3. Mesial View				
4. Distal View				
5. Incisal/ Occlusal View				

Self Evaluation Rating = $\dfrac{\text{points received}}{\text{points possible}}$ = _____ = _____ %

INSTRUCTOR EVALUATION RATING

FIVE VIEWS	Clearly Drawn	Accurate Sizing	General Features Included	Specific Features Included
1. Facial View				
2. Lingual View				
3. Mesial View				
4. Distal View				
5. Incisal/ Occlusal View				

Instructor Evaluation Rating = $\dfrac{\text{points received}}{\text{points possible}}$ = _____ = _____ %

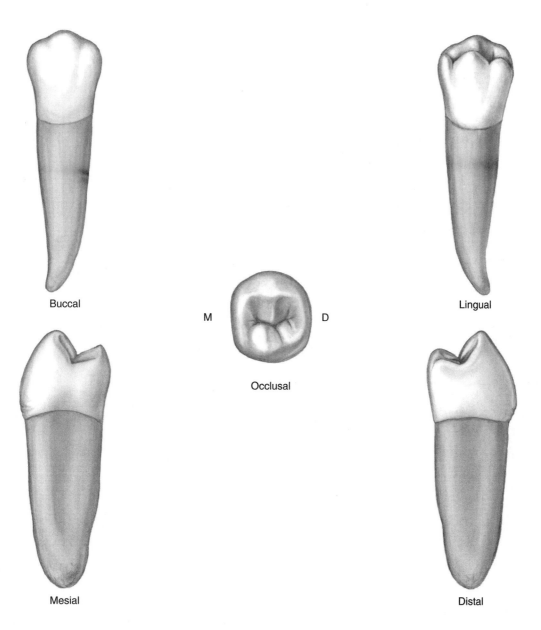

Buccal

Lingual

M   D

Occlusal

Mesial

Distal

Various Views of a Permanent Mandibular Right Second Premolar

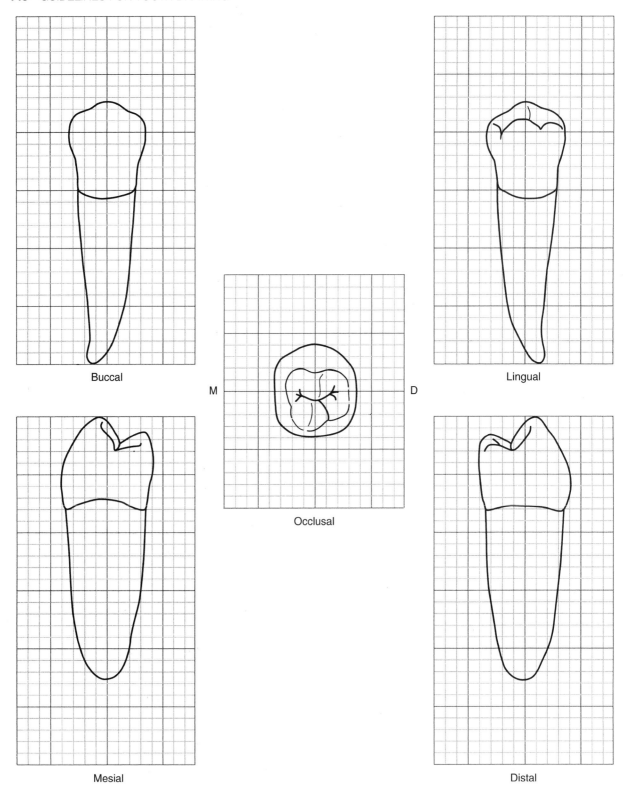

Buccal

M

D

Occlusal

Lingual

Mesial

Distal

Various Outline Views of a Permanent Mandibular Right Second Premolar

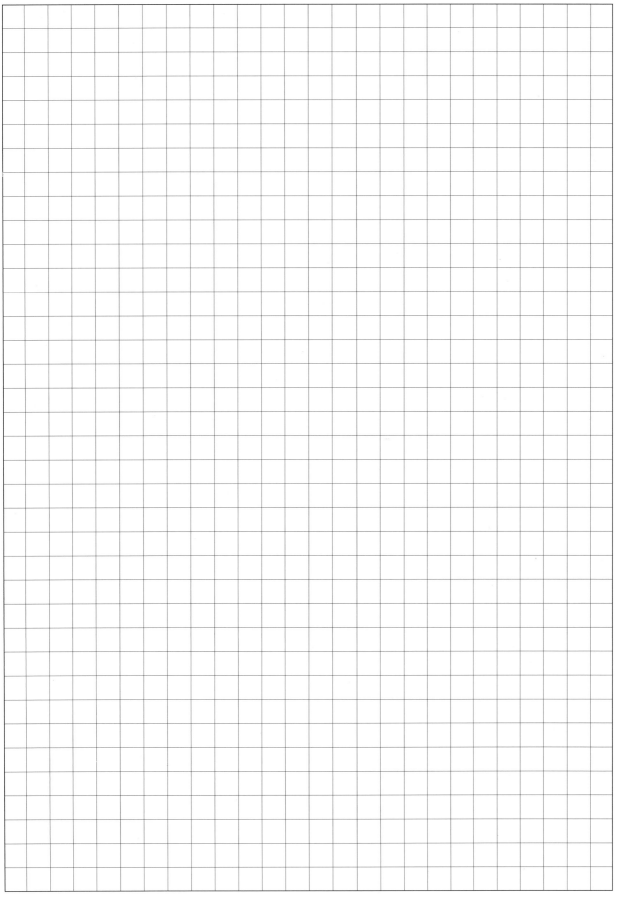

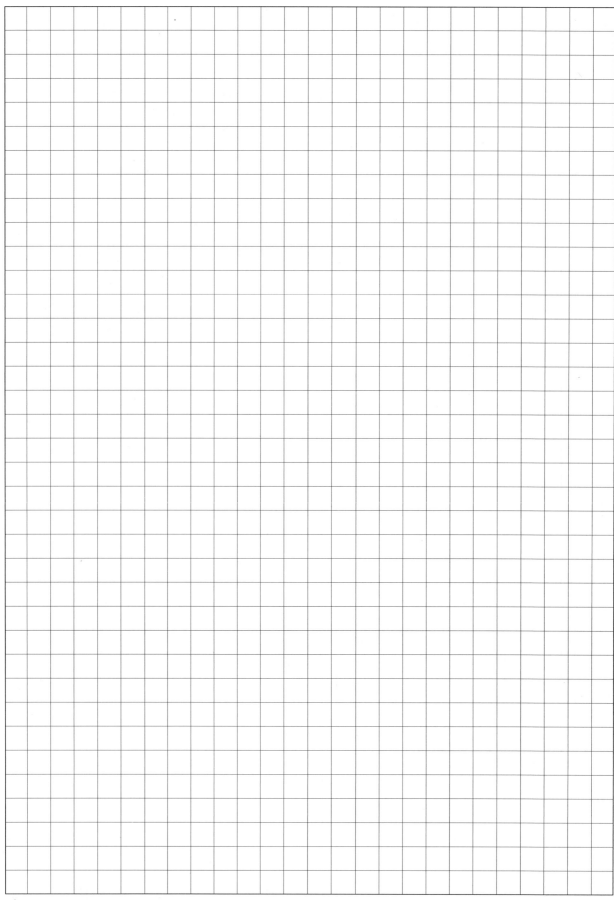

DIMENSIONS OF PERMANENT MANDIBULAR SECOND PREMOLAR*

Cervico-incisal Length of Crown	8.0
Length of Root	14.5
Mesiodistal Diameter of Crown	7.0
Mesiodistal Diameter at CEJ	5.0
Buccolingual Diameter	8.0
Buccolingual Diameter at CEJ	7.0
Curvature of CEJ—Mesial	1.0
Curvature of CEJ—Distal	0.0

*Information adapted from Ash MM, Nelson SJ: *Wheeler's Dental Anatomy, Physiology and Occlusion*, ed 8, WB Saunders, Philadelphia, 2003.

CHECKLIST FOR PERMANENT MANDIBULAR SECOND PREMOLAR

Features Noted	Features Present
Crown Features	
Usually three cusps present with buccal ridge	
Occlusal table with marginal ridges and cusps, with tips, ridges, inclined planes, and grooves (usually Y groove pattern with increased supplemental grooves), fossae, pits	
Distal marginal ridge more cervically located, so more occlusal surface visible from distal view	
Mesial and distal contact is just cervical to the junction of occlusal and middle thirds	
Root Features	
Single rooted	
Proximal root concavities	

Name _____   Tooth Number/Name _____

Date _____   Instructor Rating _____

DRAWING EVALUATION CHECKLIST

RATING SCALE
Fully Correct = 2 points   Major Error = 0 points
Minor Error = 1 point   Note: NA (non-appropriate)

SELF EVALUATION RATING

FIVE VIEWS	Clearly Drawn	Accurate Sizing	General Features Included	Specific Features Included
1. Facial View				
2. Lingual View				
3. Mesial View				
4. Distal View				
5. Incisal/ Occlusal View				

$$\text{Self Evaluation Rating} = \frac{\text{points received}}{\text{points possible}} = \underline{\hspace{3cm}} = \underline{\hspace{3cm}} \%$$

INSTRUCTOR EVALUATION RATING

FIVE VIEWS	Clearly Drawn	Accurate Sizing	General Features Included	Specific Features Included
1. Facial View				
2. Lingual View				
3. Mesial View				
4. Distal View				
5. Incisal/ Occlusal View				

$$\text{Instructor Evaluation Rating} = \frac{\text{points received}}{\text{points possible}} = \underline{\hspace{3cm}} = \underline{\hspace{3cm}} \%$$

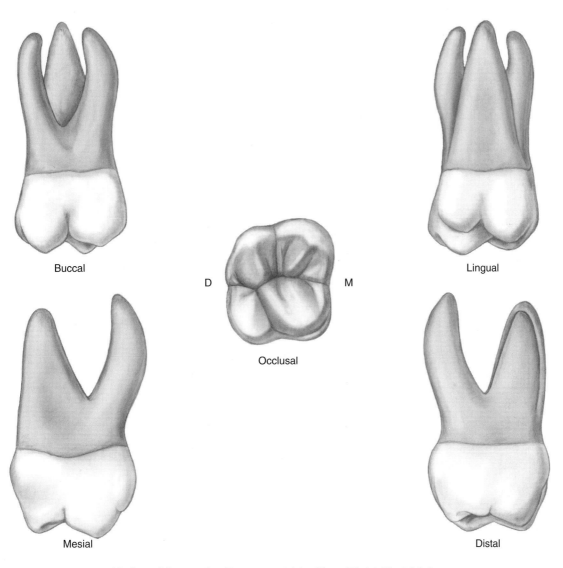

Buccal

Lingual

D   M

Occlusal

Mesial

Distal

Various Views of a Permanent Maxillary Right First Molar

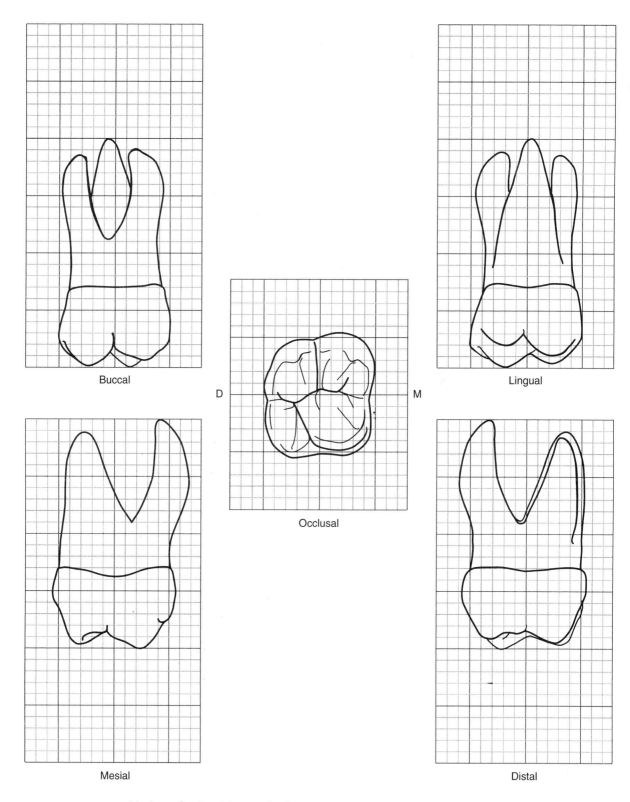

Buccal

Lingual

D   M

Occlusal

Mesial

Distal

Various Outline Views of a Permanent Maxillary Right First Molar

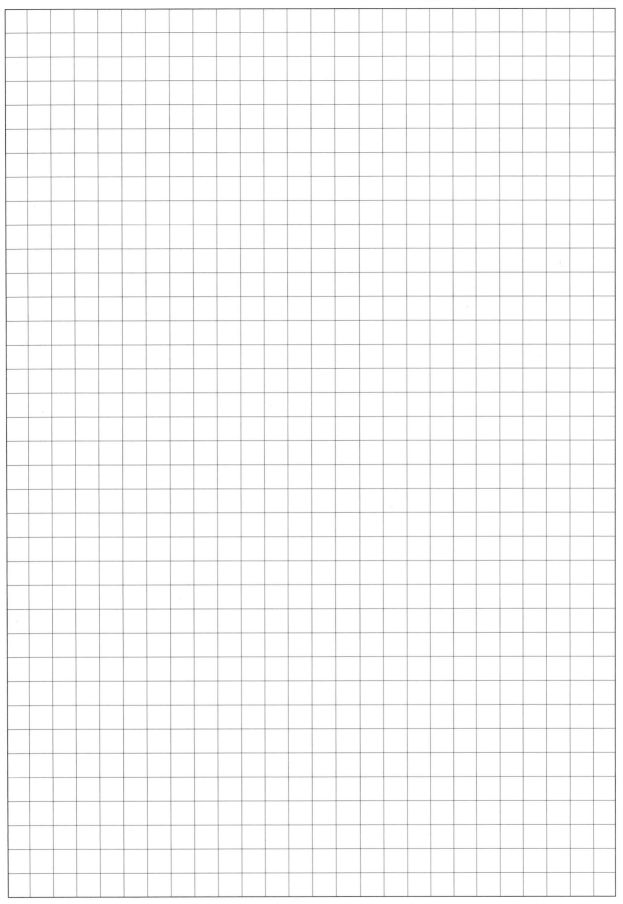

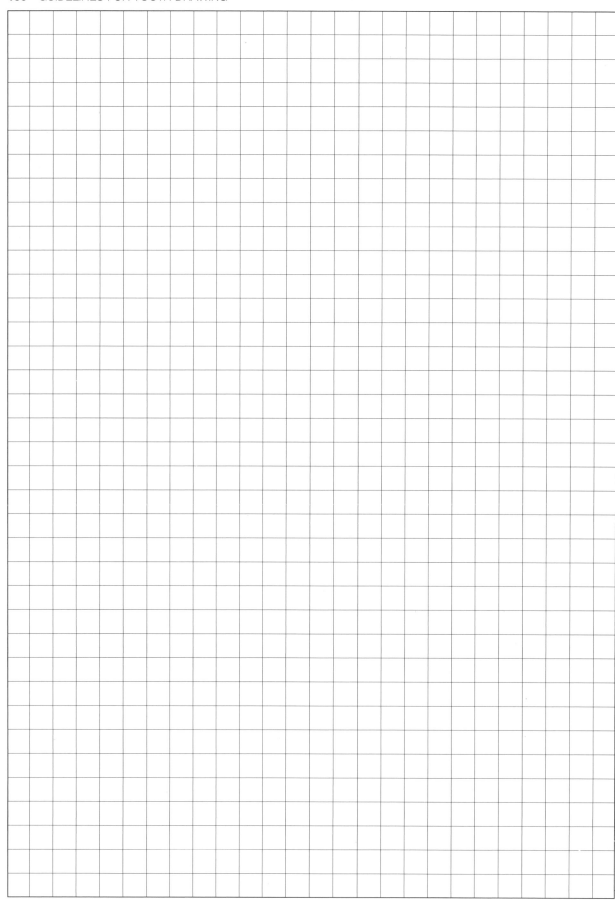

DIMENSIONS OF PERMANENT MAXILLARY FIRST MOLAR*

Cervico-incisal Length of Crown	Buccal:	7.0	Lingual:	6.0
Length of Root	Buccal:	12	Lingual:	13
Mesiodistal Diameter of Crown		10.0		
Mesiodistal Diameter at CEJ		8.0		
Buccolingual Diameter		11.0		
Buccolingual Diameter at CEJ		10.0		
Curvature of CEJ—Mesial		1.0		
Curvature of CEJ—Distal		0.0		

*Information adapted from Ash MM, Nelson SJ: *Wheeler's Dental Anatomy, Physiology and Occlusion*, ed 8, WB Saunders, Philadelphia, 2003.

CHECKLIST FOR PERMANENT MAXILLARY FIRST MOLAR

Features Noted	Features Present
Crown Features	
Four major cusps, with buccal cusps almost equal in height and fifth minor cusp of Carabelli associated with mesiolingual cusp and groove	
Buccal cervical ridge	
Mesiolingual cusp outline longer and larger, but not as sharp as distolingual cusp	
Occlusal table with prominent oblique ridge, marginal ridges and cusps, with tips, ridges, inclined planes, and grooves, fossae, pits	
Mesial contact is at junction of occlusal and middle thirds	
Distal contact at middle third	
Root Features	
Trifurcated roots, with furcations, root trunks and root concavities	
Divergent roots with furcations well-removed from the CEJ	

Name _____   Tooth Number/Name _____

Date _____   Instructor Rating _____

DRAWING EVALUATION CHECKLIST

RATING SCALE

Fully Correct = 2 points   Major Error = 0 points
Minor Error = 1 point   Note: NA (non-appropriate)

SELF EVALUATION RATING

FIVE VIEWS	Clearly Drawn	Accurate Sizing	General Features Included	Specific Features Included
1. Facial View				
2. Lingual View				
3. Mesial View				
4. Distal View				
5. Incisal/ Occlusal View				

$$\text{Self Evaluation Rating} = \frac{\text{points received}}{\text{points possible}} = \underline{\hspace{2cm}} = \underline{\hspace{2cm}} \%$$

INSTRUCTOR EVALUATION RATING

FIVE VIEWS	Clearly Drawn	Accurate Sizing	General Features Included	Specific Features Included
1. Facial View				
2. Lingual View				
3. Mesial View				
4. Distal View				
5. Incisal/ Occlusal View				

$$\text{Instructor Evaluation Rating} = \frac{\text{points received}}{\text{points possible}} = \underline{\hspace{2cm}} = \underline{\hspace{2cm}} \%$$

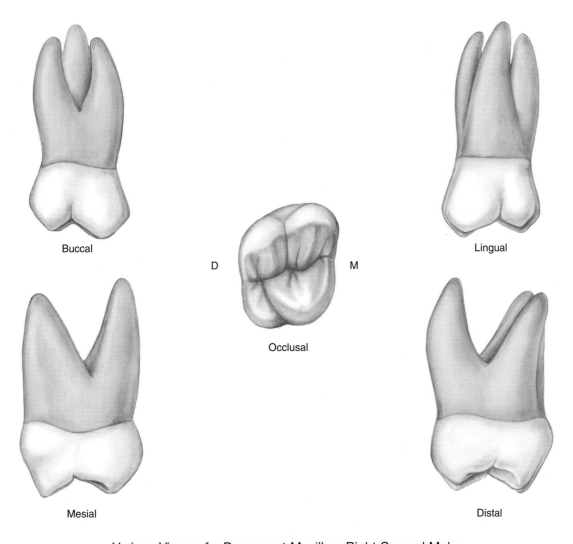

Buccal

Lingual

D   M

Occlusal

Mesial

Distal

Various Views of a Permanent Maxillary Right Second Molar

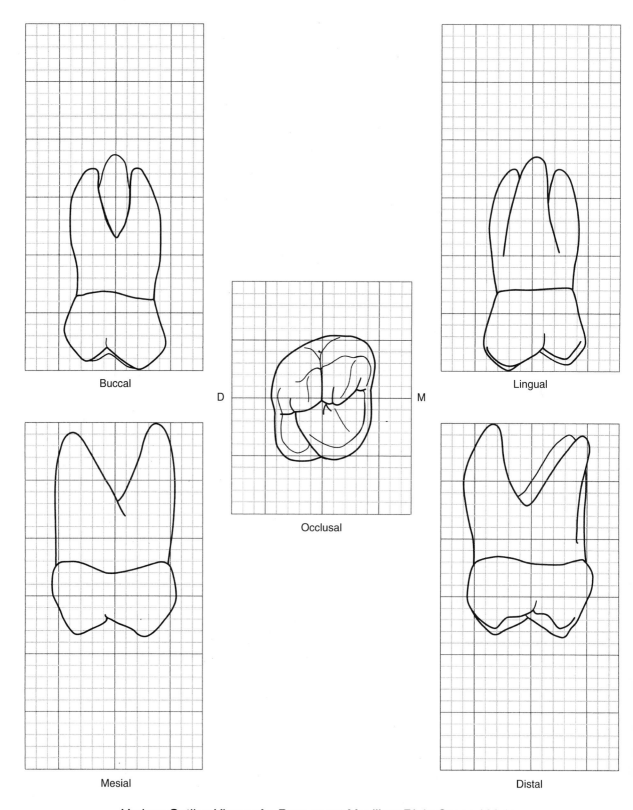

Buccal

Lingual

D — M

Occlusal

Mesial

Distal

Various Outline Views of a Permanent Maxillary Right Second Molar

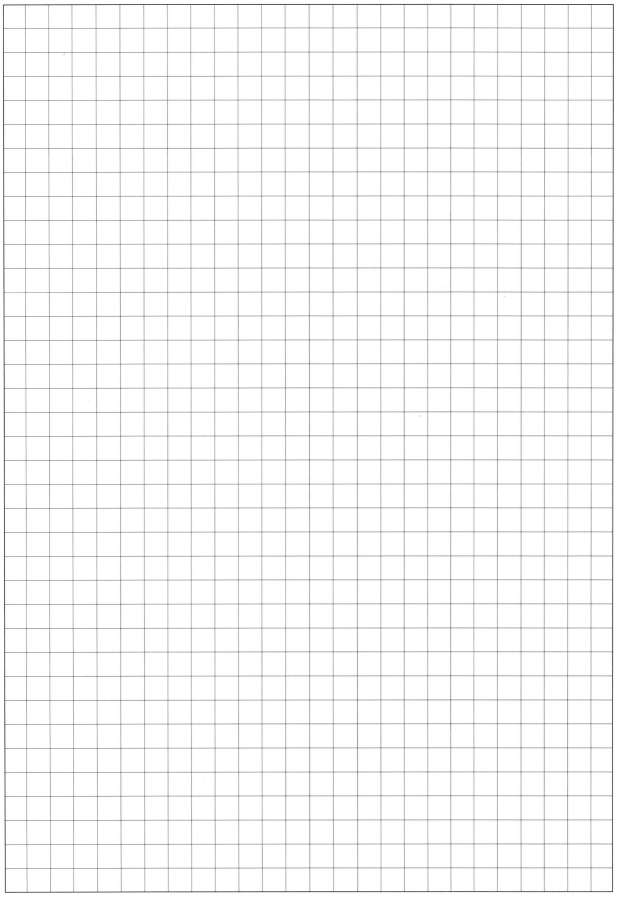

DIMENSIONS OF PERMANENT MAXILLARY SECOND MOLAR*

Cervico-incisal Length of Crown	Buccal:	6.5	Lingual:	5.5
Length of Root	Buccal:	11	Lingual:	12
Mesiodistal Diameter of Crown	9.0			
Mesiodistal Diameter at CEJ	7.0			
Buccolingual Diameter	11.0			
Buccolingual Diameter at CEJ	10.0			
Curvature of CEJ -Mesial	1.0			
Curvature of CEJ -Distal	0.0			

*Information adapted from Ash MM, Nelson SJ: *Wheeler's Dental Anatomy, Physiology and Occlusion*, ed 8, WB Saunders, Philadelphia, 2003.

CHECKLIST FOR PERMANENT MAXILLARY SECOND MOLAR

Features Noted	Features Present
Crown Features	
Four cusps usually	
Buccal cervical ridge	
Mesiobuccal cusp longer than distobuccal cusp. Distolingual cusp usually smaller	
Occlusal table with less prominent oblique ridge, marginal ridges and cusps, with tips, ridges, inclined planes, and grooves, fossae, pits	
Mesial contact at middle third	
Distal contact at middle third	
Root Features	
Trifurcated roots, with furcations, root trunks and root concavities	
Less divergent roots	

Name _____   Tooth Number/Name _____

Date _____   Instructor Rating _____

DRAWING EVALUATION CHECKLIST

RATING SCALE

Fully Correct = 2 points   Major Error = 0 points
Minor Error = 1 point   Note: NA (non-appropriate)

SELF EVALUATION RATING

FIVE VIEWS	Clearly Drawn	Accurate Sizing	General Features Included	Specific Features Included
1. Facial View				
2. Lingual View				
3. Mesial View				
4. Distal View				
5. Incisal/ Occlusal View				

Self Evaluation Rating = $\dfrac{\text{points received}}{\text{points possible}}$ = _____ = _____ %

INSTRUCTOR EVALUATION RATING

FIVE VIEWS	Clearly Drawn	Accurate Sizing	General Features Included	Specific Features Included
1. Facial View				
2. Lingual View				
3. Mesial View				
4. Distal View				
5. Incisal/ Occlusal View				

Instructor Evaluation Rating = $\dfrac{\text{points received}}{\text{points possible}}$ = _____ = _____ %

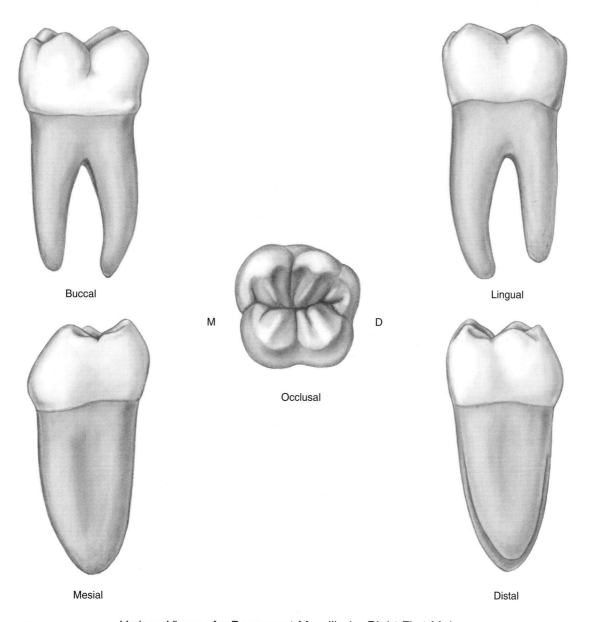

Buccal

Lingual

M

D

Occlusal

Mesial

Distal

Various Views of a Permanent Mandibular Right First Molar

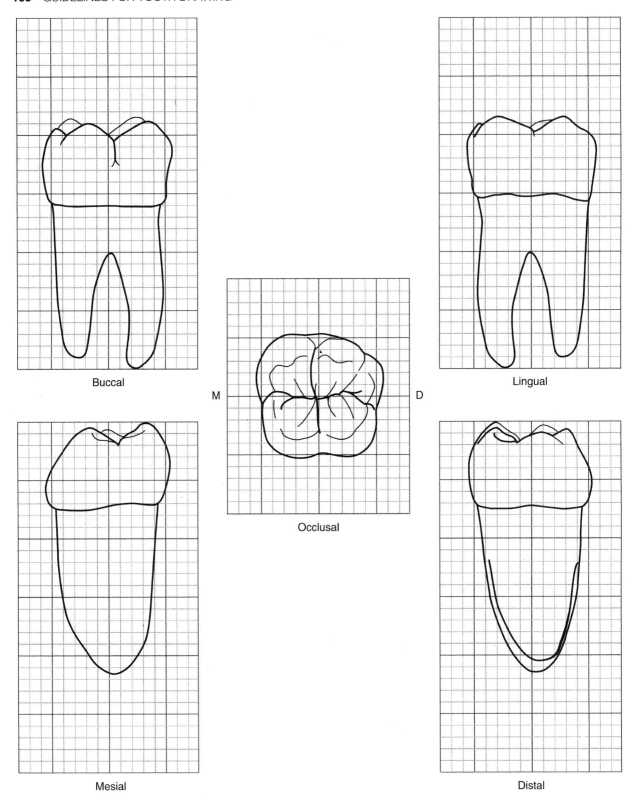

Buccal

Lingual

M   D

Occlusal

Mesial

Distal

Various Outline Views of a Permanent Mandibular Right First Molar

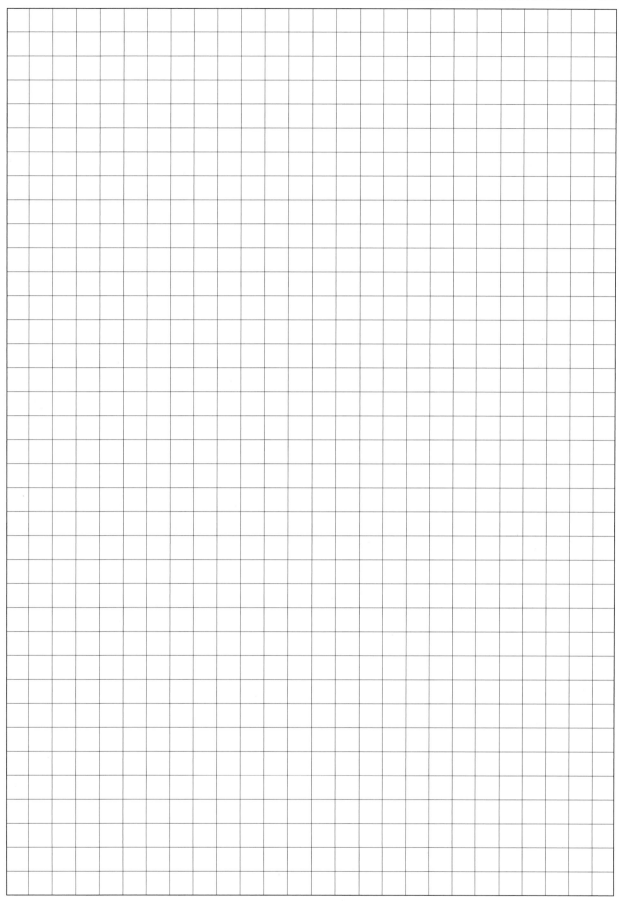

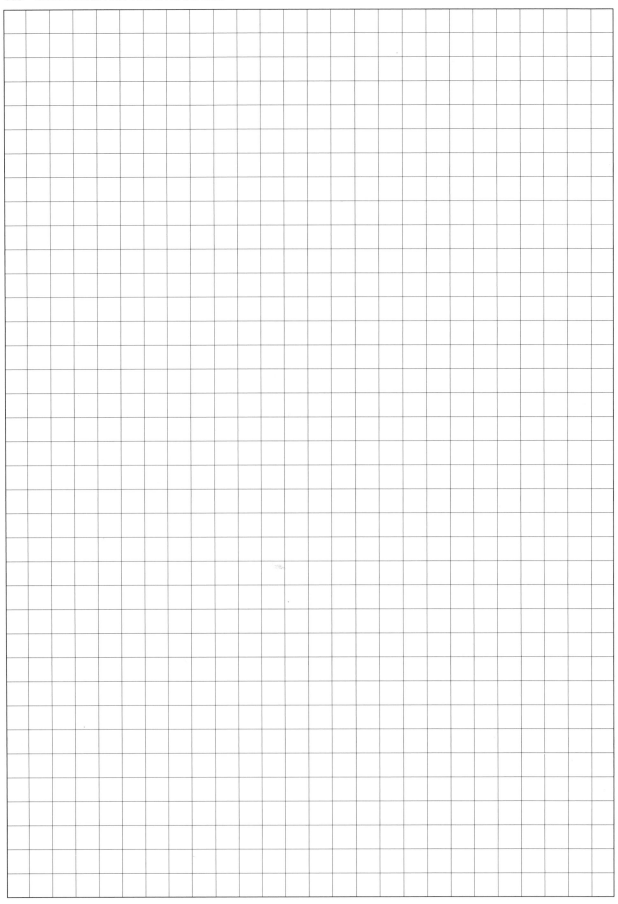

DIMENSIONS OF PERMANENT MANDIBULAR FIRST MOLAR*

Cervico-incisal Length of Crown	7.5
Length of Root	14.0
Mesiodistal Diameter of Crown	11.0
Mesiodistal Diameter at CEJ	9.0
Buccolingual Diameter	10.5
Buccolingual Diameter at CEJ	9.0
Curvature of CEJ—Mesial	1.0
Curvature of CEJ—Distal	0.0

*Information adapted from Ash MM, Nelson SJ: *Wheeler's Dental Anatomy, Physiology and Occlusion*, ed 8, WB Saunders, Philadelphia, 2003.

CHECKLIST FOR PERMANENT MANDIBULAR FIRST MOLAR

Features Noted	Features Present
Crown Features	
Five cusps with 'Y'-shaped groove pattern and with buccal groove	
Buccal cervical ridge	
Distal cusp is smallest	
Occlusal table with marginal ridges and cusps, with tips, ridges, inclined planes, and grooves, fossae, pits	
Mesial and distal contact is at junction of occlusal and middle thirds	
Root Features	
Bifurcated roots, with furcations, root trunks, and root concavities	
Divergent roots with furcations well removed from the CEJ	

Name _____   Tooth Number/Name _____

Date _____   Instructor Rating _____

DRAWING EVALUATION CHECKLIST

RATING SCALE

Fully Correct = 2 points   Major Error = 0 points
Minor Error = 1 point   Note: NA (non-appropriate)

SELF EVALUATION RATING

FIVE VIEWS	Clearly Drawn	Accurate Sizing	General Features Included	Specific Features Included
1. Facial View				
2. Lingual View				
3. Mesial View				
4. Distal View				
5. Incisal/ Occlusal View				

$$\text{Self Evaluation Rating} = \frac{\text{points received}}{\text{points possible}} = \underline{\hspace{3cm}} = \underline{\hspace{3cm}} \%$$

INSTRUCTOR EVALUATION RATING

FIVE VIEWS	Clearly Drawn	Accurate Sizing	General Features Included	Specific Features Included
1. Facial View				
2. Lingual View				
3. Mesial View				
4. Distal View				
5. Incisal/ Occlusal View				

$$\text{Instructor Evaluation Rating} = \frac{\text{points received}}{\text{points possible}} = \underline{\hspace{3cm}} = \underline{\hspace{3cm}} \%$$

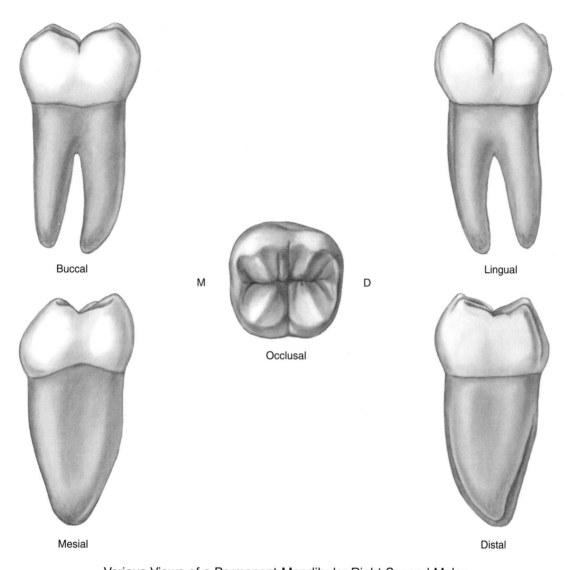

Buccal

Lingual

M

D

Occlusal

Mesial

Distal

Various Views of a Permanent Mandibular Right Second Molar

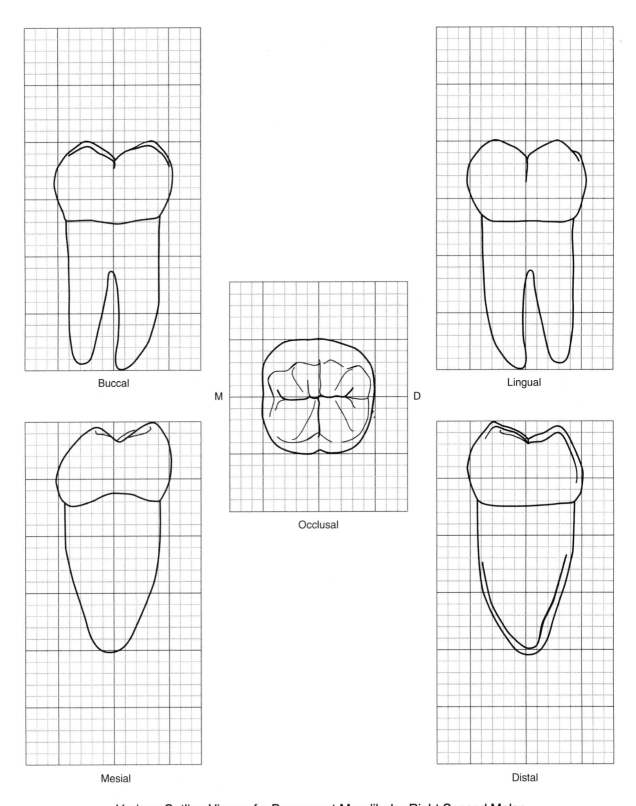

Buccal

Lingual

M   D

Occlusal

Mesial

Distal

Various Outline Views of a Permanent Mandibular Right Second Molar

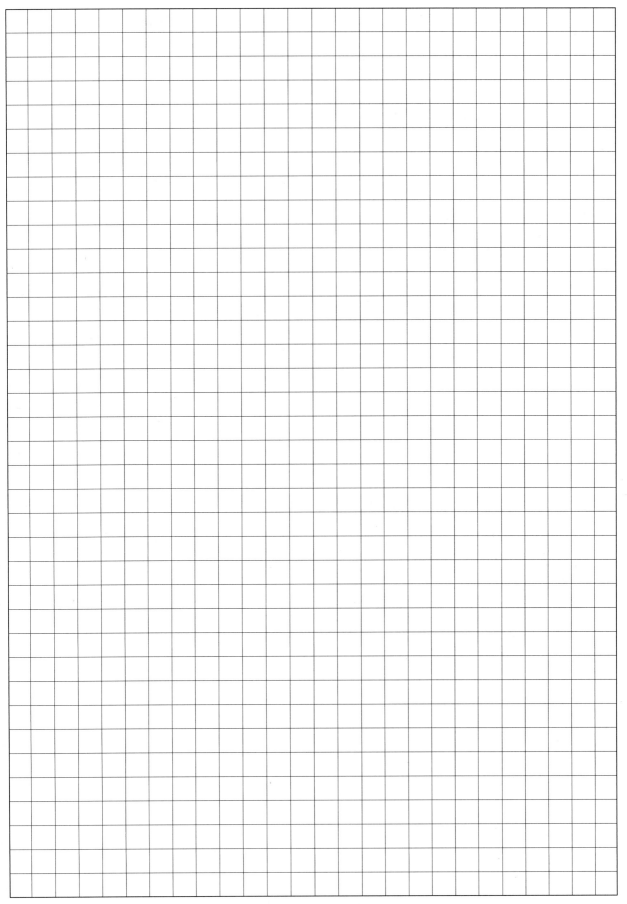

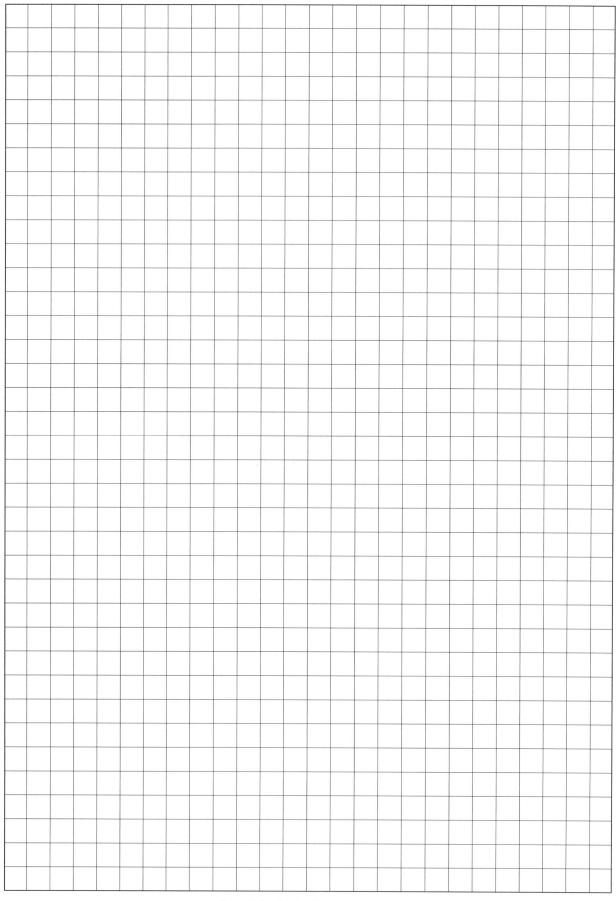

DIMENSIONS OF PERMANENT MANDIBULAR SECOND MOLAR*

Cervico-incisal Length of Crown	7.0
Length of Root	13.0
Mesiodistal Diameter of Crown	10.5
Mesiodistal Diameter at CEJ	8.0
Buccolingual Diameter	10.0
Buccolingual Diameter at CEJ	9.0
Curvature of CEJ—Mesial	1.0
Curvature of CEJ—Distal	0.0

*Information adapted from Ash MM, Nelson SJ: *Wheeler's Dental Anatomy, Physiology and Occlusion,* ed 8, WB Saunders, Philadelphia, 2003.

CHECKLIST FOR PERMANENT MANDIBULAR SECOND MOLAR

Features Noted	Features Present
Crown Features	
Four cusps with cross-shaped groove pattern	
Buccal cervical ridge	
Wider mesial proximal surface than distal	
Occlusal table with marginal ridges and cusps, with tips, ridges, inclined planes, and grooves, fossae, pits	
Mesial and distal contact is at middle third	
Root Features	
Bifurcated roots, with furcations, root trunks and root concavities	
Less divergent roots with furcations closer to CEJ	

Name _____   Tooth Number/Name _____

Date _____   Instructor Rating _____

DRAWING EVALUATION CHECKLIST

RATING SCALE
Fully Correct = 2 points   Major Error = 0 points
Minor Error = 1 point   Note: NA (non-appropriate)

SELF EVALUATION RATING

FIVE VIEWS	Clearly Drawn	Accurate Sizing	General Features Included	Specific Features Included
1. Facial View				
2. Lingual View				
3. Mesial View				
4. Distal View				
5. Incisal/ Occlusal View				

Self Evaluation Rating = $\dfrac{\text{points received}}{\text{points possible}}$ = _____ = _____ %

INSTRUCTOR EVALUATION RATING

FIVE VIEWS	Clearly Drawn	Accurate Sizing	General Features Included	Specific Features Included
1. Facial View				
2. Lingual View				
3. Mesial View				
4. Distal View				
5. Incisal/ Occlusal View				

Instructor Evaluation Rating = $\dfrac{\text{points received}}{\text{points possible}}$ = _____ = _____ %

INFECTION CONTROL FOR EXTRACTED TEETH: GUIDELINES AND TECHNIQUE

Guidelines

The use of extracted human teeth in the study of dental anatomy is a valuable addition to the analysis of plastic or plaster teeth. Extracted teeth provide a more realistic form of the anatomy of the tooth; they have more clearly formed cusps, ridges, fossae, and pits. Variations of the ideal tooth form can also be seen by the student. Extracted teeth can also provide the student with the opportunity to view relatively rare dental anomalies. Although no cases of disease transmitted by extracted teeth have been reported, sterilization of teeth used in the teaching laboratory should be a concern. However, all dental personnel who collect and inspect extracted teeth should adhere to the infection control procedures.

The Occupational Safety and Health Administration (OSHA) recommends that "extracted teeth be subject to the containerization and labeling provisions of the bloodborne standard." The Centers for Disease Control (CDC) guidelines (1993/2002) state that extracted teeth should be collected in clearly marked and "securely sealed specimen container" (wide-mouthed jar) with a 10 percent (diluted 1:10 with tap water) solution of common household bleach (sodium hypochlorite). The guidelines then specify the use of personal protective equipment when teeth are handled during preparation. New studies show that teeth also can be soaked in a solution of 10 percent formalin for one week, if desired. Because of the risk of mercury contamination during tooth preparation, teeth with amalgam cannot be saved or sterilized for viewing. A documented technique for the infection control of extracted teeth has been recently updated.[*]

Infection Control for Extracted Teeth

1. Use gloves, mask, and protective eyewear during preparation of the teeth.

2. Open collection jars, and pour off bleach solution into disposal jars, replacing it with a new 10-percent bleach solution. The old solution should be left standing for at least 30 minutes in the disposal jar and then poured into the sewer.

3. Place collected teeth on several layers of paper towels on a tray to protect desk tops. Discard collection jars and lids in any trash receptacle.

4. Separate the teeth, and place any teeth to be discard (such as those with amalgamrestorations) into a wide-mouthed jar with new 10-percent bleach solution. These teeth and jars are then discarded in any trash receptacle after 30 minutes.

5. Place remaining teeth into clear zipper-lock plastic bag with a new 10-percent bleach solution. Place closed bag in an ultrasonic for 30 minutes. Solution from the bag is poured down the sewer.

6. Teeth should be covered with a wet paper towel to maintain moisture. Place teeth in plastic autoclave bags, and tape them closed. Autoclave teeth for 40 minutes at 240 degrees F and 20 psi. Discard paper towels, plastic bag, and gloves in the biohazard waste receptacle. Spray tray with germicidal detergent, and allow to dry.

7. Place autoclaved teeth into clear wide-mouthed jars so that teeth can be viewed and then removed with cotton pliers. Jars are labeled (according to OSHA standards) and then filled with 0.2 % thymol solution. Store the teeth under the solution at all times so that they will not dry out and crack.

* Technique is modified and permission granted by original author, Dr. Thomas M. Schulein, DDS, Associate Professor, University of Iowa, Iowa City, IA (*Journal of Dental Education* 1994, 58:6). The technique has been updated from a research study done by Dominici JT, Eleazer PD, Clark SJ, Staat RH, Scheetz JP: Disinfection/sterilization of extracted teeth for dental student use (*Journal of Dental Education* 2001.65: 11). The purpose of this study was to determine the effectiveness of different sterilization/disinfection methods for extracted human teeth that were 100% effective in preventing growth by using *Bacillus stearothermophilus,* a bacteria resistant to heat and frequently used to test sterilizers.

8. As teeth are needed, they can be removed from the jars with cotton pliers and rinsed with tap water, soaked in a container of tap water, and rinsed again. Teeth can be safely handled with ungloved hands. There is no need to pretreat these teeth with thymol solutions before discarding them into the sewer.

Selected References and Additional Resources

CDC: Recommended infection control practices for dentistry, 1993. *MMWR* 1993;42(No. RR-8):1-12. www.cdc.gov/OralHealth/infection_control/faq/extracted_teeth.htm

Cuny E, Carpenter W. Extracted teeth: decontamination, disposal and use. *CDA J* 1997;25(11):801-4.

Pantera EA, and Schuster GS. Sterilization of extracted human teeth. *J Dent Educ* 1990;54:283-285.

Parsell DE, Stewart BM, Barker JR, Nick TG, Karnes L, and Johnson RB. The effect of steam sterilization on the physical properties and perceived cutting characteristics of extracted teeth. *J Dent Educ* 1998;62:260-263.

Schulein TM. Infection control for extracted teeth in the teaching laboratory. *J Dent Educ* 1994;58:411-413.

Tate WH, White RR. Disinfection of human teeth for educational purposes. *J Dent Educ* 1991;55:583-5.

US Department of Labor Occupational Safety and Health Administration. Occupational exposure to bloodborne pathogens; final rule. CFR part 1910.1030. *Federal Register*, 1991; 56:64004-182.

US Department of Labor Occupational Safety and Health Administration. Enforcement procedures for the Occupational Exposure to Bloodborne Pathogens *CPL* 2-2.69; November 27, 2001.

OCCLUSAL EVALUATION

Supplies Needed

The dental professional will need the following supplies for an initial occlusal evaluation of a permanent dentition: dental chair and light, mirror, explorer, probe, hand mirror, articulating paper, floss, and an occlusal evaluation form. Explanations of the reasons for taking an occlusal evaluation and how it relates to dental treatment, as well as the terms used in this evaluation, are located in the associated textbook. In many dental offices the occlusal evaluation is a part of the periodontal evaluation.

Occlusal History and Extraoral and Intraoral Findings

Before performing an occlusal evaluation, take notes on the **occlusal history** of your patient. Note in the chart any removable prostheses (flippers, retainers, night and sports guards, and partial and/or complete dentures), and have the patient keep them in during the evaluation if they are worn regularly. Record any occlusal complaints, habits, and applicable physical or psychological findings from the patient or health questionnaire that may be pertinent to the patient's occlusal history. Note these findings under occlusal history.

Additionally, note any information found during an **extraoral examination** that may be pertinent to the patient's occlusion. This includes any facial asymmetries, loss of vertical dimension, mandibular deviation upon opening, and temporomandibular disorder symptoms. Also note any information found during an **intraoral examination** that may be pertinent to the patient's occlusion. Note any **attrition** of the dentition, and record the location and amount involved in the area provided on the chart. Finally, note any **mobility** of the dentition by circling the involved teeth in red opposite the mobility section.

Record any **sensitivity** to thermal changes or percussion (gentle tapping). Record any deviations in the **intra-arch form or alignment,** such as loss of contact, plunging cusps, crossbites, and any arch collapse. Note also any missing, rotated, supererupted, or drifted or fractured teeth. Changes in the midline of the two dentitions should be noted also. Note these items related to intra-arch findings in the areas listed on the chart.

Finally, record any pertinent information from a **radiographic examination** of the dentition, such as amount of bone support, alterations of the periodontal ligament, root resorption, no-vital and fixed prosthetic teeth, as well as veneers and crowns. Record these findings in the area listed as the radiographic examination.

Achieving Centric Relation and Patient/Clinician Positioning

For the dental professional to evaluate the occlusion of a patient, the patient must be first in centric relation. **Centric relation (CR)** is the end point of closure of the mandible in which the mandible is in the most retruded position. Centric relation is used as a baseline for an occlusal evaluation.

To achieve centric relation, the patient first is placed in an upright position. The patient should be relaxed, looking straight ahead, lips parted. The clinician should be sitting or standing in front and to the side of the patient. The clinician's thumb should be placed against the outside of the chin, with the fingers placed under the inferior border of the mandible to alternately lift and loosen the mandible. The clinician must then establish the hinge movement of the mandible by gently arcing the mandible with the fingers in a closing and opening manner several times. Then, the loosened mandible is guided into closure, where the mandible is placed in its most retruded position.

Determining Angle's Classification of Malocclusion

Once the patient is in centric relation, determine **Angle's classification of malocclusion** to determine the form of the patient's dentition. Most cases can be placed into three main classes on the basis of the position of the permanent maxillary first molar relative to the mandibular first molar. The position of the canines must be noted also. Additionally, any subgroups within the classification must be noted. The classification is recorded in the area on the chart labeled *Angle's classification*. A tendency to any type of malocclusion can be noted using the molar relationship (less than the width of a premolar).

Measuring Overjet

With the patient maintained in centric relation, **overjet** or horizontal overlap between the two arches is measured in millimeters with the tip of the periodontal probe. The probe is placed at a right angle to the labial surface of a mandibular incisor at the base of the of the incisal edge of a maxillary incisor. The measurement is taken from the labial surface of the mandibular incisor to the lingual surface of the maxillary incisor. Note that the labiolingual width of the maxillary incisor is not included in the measurement. The overjet is recorded in the chart in the area labeled *overjet*.

Measuring Overbite

Overbite, or vertical overlap between the two arches, is measured in millimeters with the tip of the periodontal probe after the patient is placed in centric relation. The probe is placed on the incisal edge of the maxillary incisor at right angles to the mandibular incisor. As the patient opens the mouth or depresses the jaws, the probe is then placed vertically against the mandibular incisor to measure the distance to the incisal edge of the mandibular incisor. The overbite is recorded in the chart in the area labeled *overbite*.

Checking for Interocclusal Clearance

Allow the patient to rest while checking for **interocclusal clearance**, the space when the mandible is at rest. In this rest position, an average space of 2 to 3 millimeterscan be noted between the masticatory surfaces of the maxillary and mandibular teeth. Thus failure of a patient to assume this position when the jaws are not at work may mean the patient is temporarily tense or has parafunctional habits such as clenching or grinding (bruxism). Interocclusal clearance is measured in millimeters and recorded in the area for it on the chart. If no interocclusal clearance is noted during mandibular rest, follow-up questions may be necessary to ascertain any tension or parafunctional habits.

Checking for Premature Contact

After the patient relaxes for a moment, centric relation is again attained and the patient is asked where the teeth first touch during occlusion. If it is a lone tooth, the tooth is considered to be part of a **premature contact**. Articulation paper can be used to check for these premature contacts, which limit the opportunity for maximal intercuspation of the teeth. Premature contacts are recorded in the chart by circling the tooth numbers of the contacting teeth in red opposite the centric relation occlusion section.

Achieving Centric Occlusion

Next, have the patient clench the teeth together, and note the amount of slide in millimeters from their position in centric relation to their position in centric relation. **Centric occlusion (CO),** or habitual occlusion, is the voluntary position of the dentition that allows maximal contact when the teeth occlude. Record the amount of slide or shift in millimeters in the chart; the direction of the slide is also recorded (anterior, right, left, posterior). Normally, the amount of slide or shift from CR to CO is about 1 millimeter. If no slide is noted, then position of the teeth in centric relation is the same as in centric occlusion and CR = CO is circled in the chart.

Checking Lateral Occlusion

Next, the patient's occlusion in lateral deviation or excursion must be checked. Evaluation of **lateral occlusion** is made by moving the mandible to either the right or the left until the canines on that side are in **canine rise,** or cuspid rise. The clinician must support the patient's mandible with the operating hand and gently move the mandible into centric relation or even centric occlusion. Then, the clinician slowly guides the mandible to the patient's right or left until the opposing canines are edge to edge.

The side to which the mandible has been moved is the **working side**. There are two working sides noted in an occlusal evaluation: right lateral and left lateral. Before the canines come into contact on each side, other individual teeth that make contact on the working side should be noted. These **working contacts** are recorded by circling the tooth numbers of the contacting teeth in blue on the chart in the area opposite the lateral occlusion section for the appropriate side.

The other side of the arch from the working side during lateral occlusion is the **balancing side**. If any teeth make contact on the opposite or balancing side during lateral occlusion, they are recorded as a **balancing interference** and are circled in red for the appropriate side. If **group function,** where most of the entire posterior quadrant functions during lateral occlusion, is present, it should be recorded by circling the tooth numbers of the involved group of teeth in blue on the chart opposite the lateral occlusion section for the appropriate side.

Do not allow patients to move freely into lateral deviation because they may choose a convenience path to bypass an interference. For further confirmation of any balancing interferences during lateral deviation, place floss across the retromolar pads extending out to the labial commissures or place articulating paper over the occlusal surfaces on the appropriate side. After guiding the patient into either right or left lateral occlusion, the clinician slips the floss or articulating paper forward, noting any points of contact.

Checking Protrusive Occlusion

Finally, the **protrusive occlusion** of the patient must be checked. With the patient's teeth in centric occlusion, the clinician supports the mandible with the operating hand. Have the patient slowly move the mandible forward so that the two dentitions are in an edge-to-edge relationship. Note any posterior/canine contacts or **balancing interferences** during protrusion, and record this information on the chart by circling the contacting teeth in red opposite the protrusive section. Also note the anterior teeth that are contact during protrusion, or the **working contacts,** by circling on the chart the tooth numbers of the contacting teeth in blue opposite the protrusive section.

For further confirmation of working contacts and any balancing interferences during protrusion, place the floss across the retromolar pads extending out to the labial commissures. Then, guide the patient into protrusive occlusion, and slip the floss forward between the teeth until resistance of contacting teeth is met.

INITIAL OCCLUSAL EXAMINATION

Patient Name _____ Chart No. _____ Date _____

Occlusal History _____

_____

Extraoral Findings _____

_____

Intraoral Findings _____

_____

Angle's Classification _____ **Molar** _____ **Canine** _____ **Subgroup**

Interocclusal Clearance _____ mm **Sensitivity** _____

Overjet _____ mm **Overbite** _____ mm **Attrition** _____

Intra-arch Form/Alignment _____

_____

Radiographic Examination _____

_____

INITIAL OCCLUSAL FINDINGS																	
Centric Relation	1	2	3	4	5	6	7	8	9	10	11	12	13	14	15	16	
Occlusion	32	31	30	29	28	27	26	25	24	23	22	21	20	19	18	17	
CR = CO	mm shift from CR to CO								anterior right left posterior								
Right Lateral	1	2	3	4	5	6	7	8	9	10	11	12	13	14	15	16	
Occlusion	32	31	30	29	28	27	26	25	24	23	22	21	20	19	18	17	
Left Lateral	1	2	3	4	5	6	7	8	9	10	11	12	13	14	15	16	
Occlusion	32	31	30	29	28	27	26	25	24	23	22	21	20	19	18	17	
Protrusive	1	2	3	4	5	6	7	8	9	10	11	12	13	14	15	16	
Occlusion	32	31	30	29	28	27	26	25	24	23	22	21	20	19	18	17	
Mobility	1	2	3	4	5	6	7	8	9	10	11	12	13	14	15	16	
	32	31	30	29	28	27	26	25	24	23	22	21	20	19	18	17	

Case
Studies

CASE STUDY 1

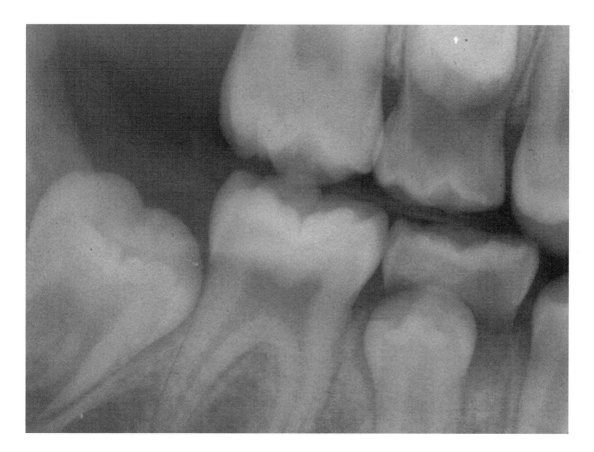

Patient Profile: Male child, age 11.

Chief Complaint: "Why do my back teeth feel real loose?"

Dental History: Patient has been to the dentist once before at age 7, and sealants were placed on all erupted permanent posterior teeth.

Medical History: None noted.

Intraoral Examination: A bite-wing radiograph was taken on both sides of the mouth. Four posterior teeth are loose, and four teeth are partially erupted.

Supplemental Notes: Inflammation is noted around loose and partially erupted teeth.

1. On which teeth were sealants placed at the last dental appointment?
   a. First molars
   b. Second molars
   c. First premolars
   d. Second premolars

2. Which partially erupted teeth may need to be sealed at the next appointment because of their risk of caries?
   a. First molars
   b. Second molars
   c. First premolars
   d. Second premolars

3. Which of the following teeth may be loose and ready to be exfoliated?
   a. #2
   b. #30
   c. T
   d. S

4. The crown of which permanent posterior tooth appears similar to the crown anatomy of one of the loose teeth?
   a. #2
   b. #30
   c. T
   d. S

5. Which of the following teeth have already been exfoliated?
   a. #2
   b. #30
   c. T
   d. S

CASE STUDY 2

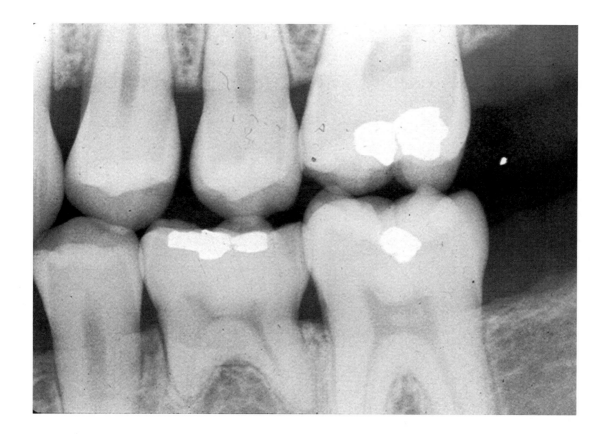

Patient Profile: Female adult, age 25.

Chief Complaint: "Why is one of my back teeth smaller than the rest?"

Dental History: Patient has a new dentist. At age 6, sealants were placed on four teeth that were later restored. Patient had four permanent posterior teeth extracted at age 13 because of extensive caries and four more at age 20 because of impaction. Her most recent dentist told her that some of her "adult" teeth were never going to erupt.

Medical History: None.

Intraoral Examination: A bite-wing radiograph was taken on both sides of the mouth. A small posterior tooth was noted on both sides of mouth.

Supplemental Notes: The patient is having difficulty with oral hygiene on her small teeth. She regularly chews sugared gum and does not live in a water-fluoridated region.

1. For which posterior tooth does the patient exhibit partial anodontia?
   a. Second premolars
   b. First molars
   c. Second molars
   d. Third molars

2. Which posterior teeth did the patient have extracted as an adolescent?
   a. Second premolars
   b. First molars
   c. Second molars
   d. Third molars

3. Which posterior teeth did the patient have extracted as a young adult?
   a. Second premolars
   b. First molars
   c. Second molars
   d. Third molars

4. Which posterior permanent teeth have been restored in the patient?
   a. Second premolars
   b. First molars
   c. Second molars
   d. Third molars

5. Of the teeth present in the patient, which of following teeth have two roots?
   a. Second premolars
   b. First molars
   c. Second molars
   d. Third molars

CASE STUDY 3

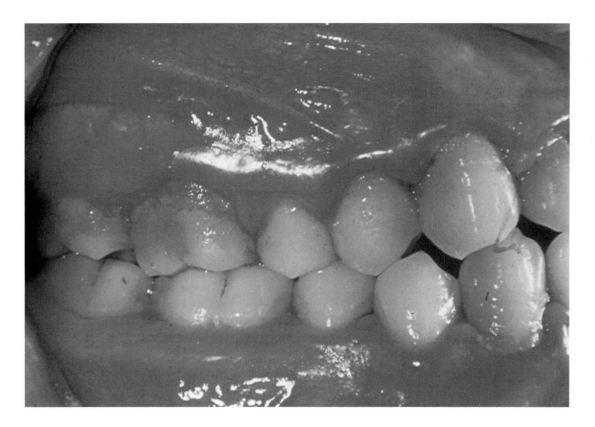

Patient Profile: Male adult, age 42.

Chief Complaint: "Why are my bottom eyeteeth sensitive at the gumline when I drink coffee?"

Dental History: Patient had orthodontics as a teenager but did not wear a retainer. Third molars were extracted at age 20. Patient grinds his teeth at night. He has not visited a dentist in 12 years. No caries were noted.

Medical History: The patient smokes and has high blood pressure.

Intraoral Examination: A clinical photograph was taken of both sides of the mouth, along with a complete set of radiographs. Moderate inflammation of the gingiva is present, with deposits noted throughout.

Supplemental Notes: Patient has always used a soft toothbrush and gargled.

1. What is Angle's Classification of the patient's posterior dentition on the right side?
   a. Class I
   b. Class II, Division I
   c. Class II, Division II
   d. Class III

2. What other occlusal notes can be made regarding the right side of the dentition?
   a. Severe crossbite
   b. Openbite
   c. Severe overjet
   d. End-to-end bite

3. What may be occurring on the patient's lower teeth to make them sensitive to hot fluids?
   a. Erosion
   b. Abfraction
   c. Pulpitis
   d. Toothbrush abrasion

4. What is the correct term for grinding the teeth?
   a. Clenching
   b. Xerostomia
   c. Bruxism
   d. Passive eruption

5. What part of the anatomy of the tooth is initially lost with grinding?
   a. Fossae
   b. Pits
   c. Fissures
   d. Cusps

CASE STUDY 4

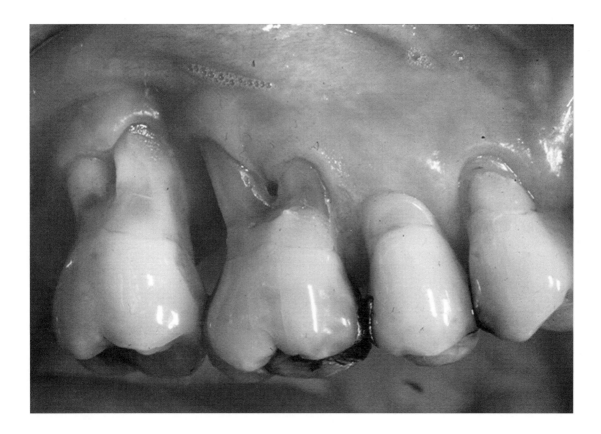

Patient Profile: Female adult, age 57.

Chief Complaint: "Why are my teeth so long?"

Dental History: Patient regularly visited the dentist until her dentist retired 15 years ago.

Medical History: None.

Intraoral Examination: A clinical photograph was taken of both sides of the mouth, along with a complete set of radiographs. Exposed roots were noted throughout, with moderate to severe bone loss. Slight bleeding and moderate mobility were observed throughout.

Supplemental Notes: Patient notes that her teeth are slightly loose.

1. What type of bone has the patient lost between the roots of her molars?
   a. Basal bone
   b. Alveolar crest bone
   c. Interdental bone
   d. Interradicular bone

2. What fiber group of the periodontal ligament was the first group to be affected by periodontal disease in this patient?
   a. Alveolar crest group
   b. Horizontal group
   c. Oblique group
   d. Apical group

3. The patient's lost cementum, alveolar bone, and periodontal ligament were a part of her:
   a. TMJ apparatus
   b. Periodontium
   c. Principal fiber group
   d. Alveolodental ligament

4. What portion of the posterior teeth was initially lost as a result of the root exposure?
   a. Predentin
   b. Secondary dentin
   c. Cellular cementum
   d. Cervical enamel

5. Which cell population has been active in removing the alveolar bone in the patient?
   a. Ameloblast
   b. Osteoclast
   c. Odotoblast
   d. Odontoclast

CASE STUDY 5

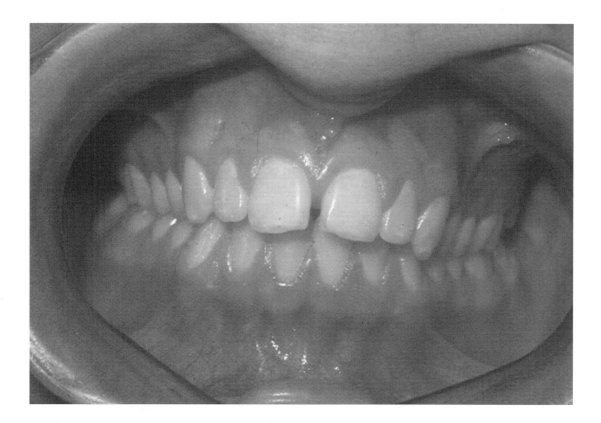

Patient Profile: Male adult, age 32.
Chief Complaint: "Why do my teeth bleed when I floss?"
Dental History: Patient has not been to the dentist in 5 years. His previous dentist told him that he needed to brush more.
Medical History: None.
Intraoral Examination: A clinical photograph was taken of both sides of the mouth, along with a complete set of radiographs. Moderate bleeding is noted but no bone loss.
Supplemental Notes: Patient does not regularly brush or floss his teeth.

1. What type of mucosa is involved in the inflammation noted in the patient?
   a. Lining mucosa
   b. Specialized mucosa
   c. Masticatory mucosa
   d. Paranasal mucosa

2. What portion of the periodontal ligament was the first to be affected in this patient?
   a. Gingival fiber group
   b. Alveolar crest group
   c. Horizontal group
   d. Oblique group

3. What is the main underlying cause of this patient's gingival bleeding when flossing?
   a. Thickening of the junctional epithelium
   b. Repair of the lamina propria's blood vessels
   c. Increased blood vessels in the lamina propria
   d. Increased collagen production around blood vessels

4. What is the name given to the patient's present periodontal condition?
   a. Active gingivitis
   b. Chronic gingivitis
   c. Active periodontitis
   d. Chronic periodontitis

5. What is the histological picture of this patient in both the epithelium and lamina propria at the dentogingival junction?
   a. Smooth interface
   b. Small numbers of white blood cells
   c. Formation of rete pegs and papillae
   d. All signs of chronic inflammation

CASE STUDY 6

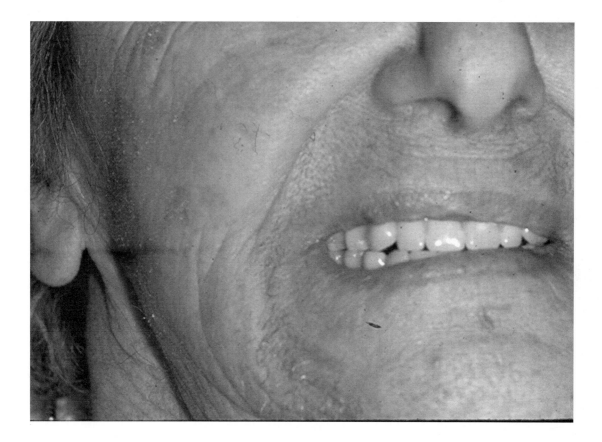

Patient Profile: Female adult, age 72.
Chief Complaint: "Why does my mouth feel sore under my dentures?"
Dental History: Patient is seeing the dentist for the first time in the nursing home.
Medical History: Patient takes antidepressants for the early stages of Alzheimer's.
Intraoral Examination: Moderate dryness is noted in mouth.
Supplemental Notes: Patient's upper and lower complete dentures do not fit comfortably.

1. What is the term for decreased salivary production?
   a. Erosion
   b. Abfraction
   c. Abrasion
   d. Xerostomia

2. Which is the largest salivary gland in the patient?
   a. Parotid
   b. Submandibular
   c. Sublingual
   d. Von Ebner's

3. What salivary gland usually produces the most saliva?
   a. Parotid
   b. Submandibular
   c. Sublingual
   d. Von Ebner's

4. What portion of the jaw bones is still completely present in this patient?
   a. Basal bone
   b. Alveolar bone
   c. Interdental bone
   d. Interradicular bone

5. The patient is experiencing diminished length of the lower third of the face; what is this called?
   a. Increase in golden proportions
   b. Loss of vertical dimension
   c. Partially edentulous state
   d. Mesial drift and supereruption

CASE STUDY 7

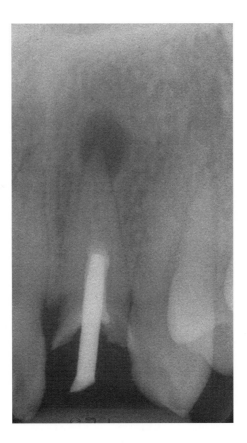

Patient Profile: Male adult, age 45.

Chief Complaint: "Can you fix my painful broken tooth?"

Dental History: When the patient was in his 20s, the affected tooth was treated with root canal surgery because of a dental anomaly. The patient experiences pain on percussion.

Medical History: None.

Intraoral Examination: A radiograph of the involved tooth was taken. An abscess at the apex of the tooth was noted.

Supplemental Notes: Patient has bad taste in the mouth.

1. What is the dental anomaly that was present in this tooth?
   a. Fusion
   b. Gemination
   c. Dens in dente
   d. Peg lateral

2. Why is the patient experiencing pain with this tooth?
   a. Secondary dentin is filling pulp chamber
   b. Inflammatory edema is pressing on nerves
   c. Inert material is extruding from the pulp
   d. Apical bone is forming at the apex

3. Why did the tooth break in the patient?
   a. Darkening of the tooth
   b. Failure at lobular division
   c. Loss of tooth vitality
   d. Placement of gutta-percha

4. What is the main path by which infection from the pulp travels to the surrounding apical periodontium and causes an abscess?
   a. Apical foramen
   b. Pulp horns
   c. Accessory canals
   d. Dentinal tubules

5. Which cell population can be called upon to produce additional pulp tissue after an injury such as the one this patient has experienced?
   a. Odontoblasts
   b. Red blood cells
   c. White blood cells
   d. Undifferentiated mesenchymal cells

CASE STUDY 8

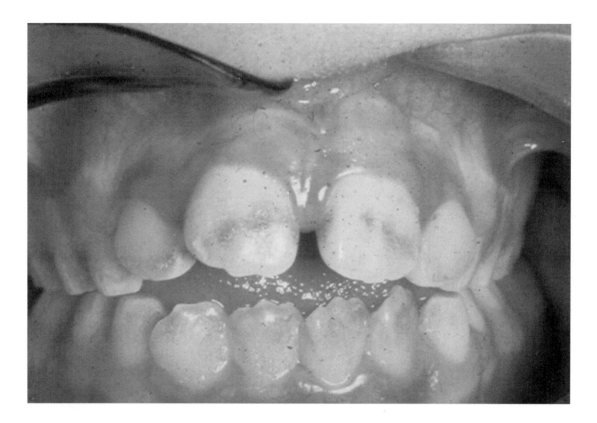

Patient Profile: Female adult, age 20.

Chief Complaint: "Can we whiten my front teeth?"

Dental History: Patient visits dentist regularly every 6 months

Medical History: None.

Intraoral Examination: Clinical photograph of dentition was taken. Patient has always had this staining of her teeth. Her previous dentist recommended full coverage crowns but said that she needed to wait until the teeth were fully erupted.

Supplemental Notes: Patient used to suck her thumb. When younger, the patient briefly lived in an area with naturally high levels of fluoride in the drinking water.

1. What is the dental disturbance that is present in the anterior teeth?
   a. Concresence
   b. Enamel dysplasia
   c. Dentinal dysplasia
   d. Chronic pulpitis

2. To cause this staining, which cell population was mainly disturbed by the high levels of fluoride?
   a. Odontoblasts
   b. Fibroblasts
   c. Ameloblasts
   d. Cementoblasts

3. During what stage(s) of tooth development does this disturbance occur?
   a. Bud stage
   b. Initiation stage
   c. Cap or bell stages
   d. Apposition and maturation stages

4. What type of staining is present in this patient?
   a. Extrinsic
   b. Intrinsic
   c. Transient
   d. Temporary

5. Because the patient has an open bite, what is also present on the incisal edges of the mandibular anterior teeth?
   a. Attrition
   b. Perikymata
   c. Mamelons
   d. Occusal table

CASE STUDY 9

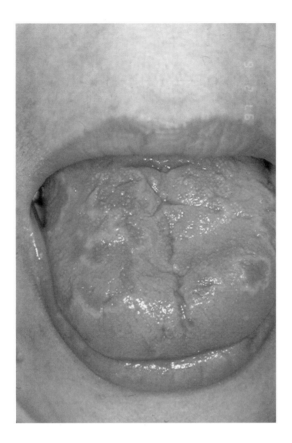

Patient Profile: Female adult, age 26.
Chief Complaint: "Why does the top of my tongue look funny?"
Dental History: The patient visits the dentist regularly. She uses an electric toothbrush.
Medical History: None.
Intraoral Examination: Clinical photograph of tongue was taken. Patient has always had this condition of the dorsal surface of the tongue. Her tongue is sore.
Supplemental Notes: The patient brushes tongue regularly as directed but does not know why.

1. What is the condition noted on the patient's dorsal surface of the tongue?
   a. Fissured tongue
   b. Central papillary atrophy
   c. Geographic tongue
   d. Burning mouth syndrome

2. What lingual papillae are involved in this tongue condition?
   a. Filiform
   b. Fugiform
   c. Circumvallate
   d. Foliate

3. What type of oral mucosa is on the dorsal surface of the tongue?
   a. Masticatory
   b. Lining
   c. Specialized
   d. Paranasal

4. What week of prenatal development does the tongue begin its specific development?
   a. First week
   b. Second week
   c. Third week
   d. Fourth week

5. The median lingual sulcus noted on the patient's tongue is a superficial demarcation of the fusion of what swellings?
   a. Lateral lingual
   b. Copula
   c. Epiglottic
   d. Tuberculum impar

CASE STUDY 10

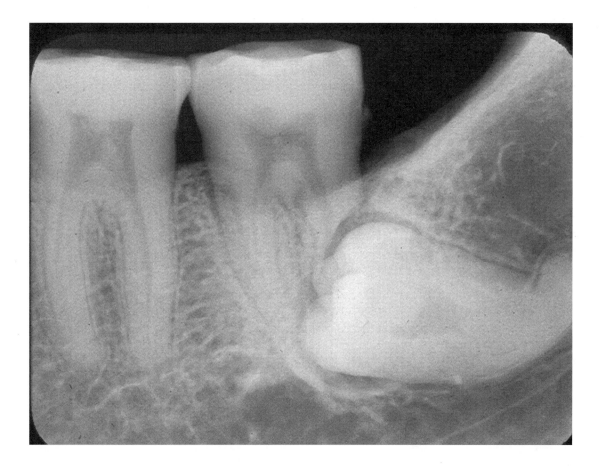

Patient Profile: Male adult, age 19.

Chief Complaint: "Why does my jaw hurt more even with my guard?"

Dental History: Patient had orthodontic treatment 8 years ago. He has a low risk of caries. He wears a night guard because of grinding of the teeth and early symptoms of temporomandibular joint disorder.

Medical History: None.

Intraoral Examination: A periapical radiograph was taken of the sore area of the jaw. No lesions in mouth were noted.

Supplemental Notes: Patient has generalized moderate attrition.

1. What is the painful condition noted on the patient's radiograph?
   a. Cyst formation
   b. Microdontia
   c. Partial anodontia
   d. Impacted third molar

2. Which of the following are features of the tooth that is causing the patient's discomfort?
   a. Three roots
   b. Four pulp horns
   c. Consistent crown form
   d. Square crown outline

3. When does the tooth that is causing the patient's discomfort usually complete its roots?
   a. 10-14 years
   b. 13-17 years
   c. 17-21 years
   d. 18-25 years

4. What are the opaque structures noted in the pulp chambers of some of the mandibular posterior teeth?
   a. Denticles
   b. Pulp stones
   c. Sialoliths
   d. Enamel pearls

5. Which structure is located on the patient's temporal bone anterior to the articular fossa of the temporomandibular joint?
   a. Joint capsule
   b. Articular eminence
   c. Synovial membrane
   d. Articulating surface of the condyle

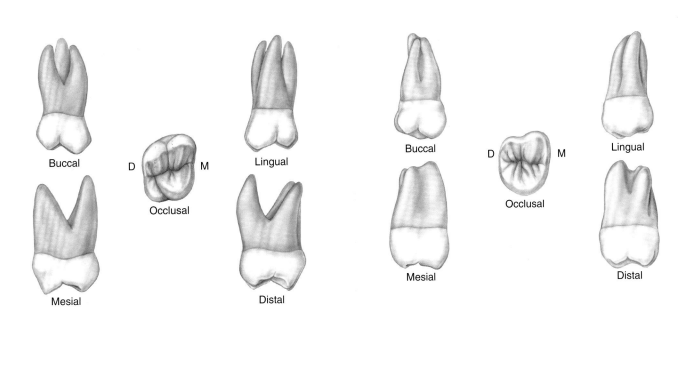

Buccal

D ⟶ M

Occlusal

Lingual

Mesial

Distal

Buccal

D ⟶ M

Occlusal

Lingual

Mesial

Distal

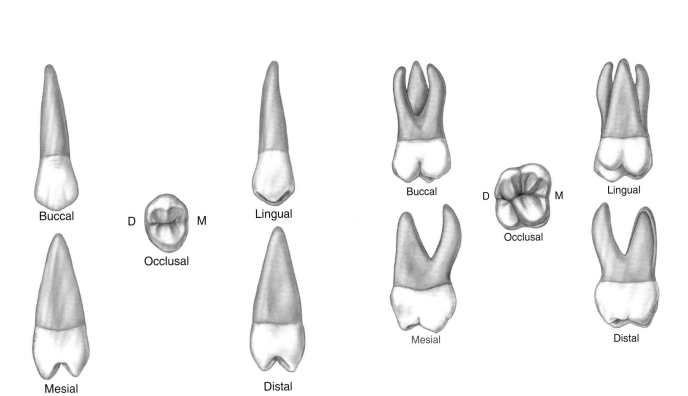

Buccal

D ⟶ M

Occlusal

Lingual

Mesial

Distal

Buccal

D ⟶ M

Occlusal

Lingual

Mesial

Distal

Maxillary Right Third Molar (Heart-shaped Occlusal Outline)

CHARACTERISTICS:

Universal Number: #1
Eruption date: 17-21 years
General crown features: Occlusal table with marginal ridges, cusps with tips, inclined planes, ridges, grooves, fossae, and pits. Buccal cervical ridge
Specific crown features: Smaller crown than second, variable in form, heart-shaped or rhomboidal crown outline, thus three or four cusps
Mesial contact: Middle third
Distal contact: None
Distinguishing right from left: Distobuccal cusp shorter than mesiobuccal cusp and roots curved distally
Root features: Usually fused roots, curving distally

Maxillary Right Second Molar (Rhombodial Crown Outline)

CHARACTERISTICS:

Universal Number: #2
Eruption date: 12-13 years
General crown features: Occlusal table with marginal ridges, cusps with tips, inclined planes, ridges, grooves, fossae, and pits. Buccal cervical ridge
Specific crown features: Smaller crown than first, heart-shaped or rhomboidal crown outline, thus three or four cusps. Oblique ridge less prominent, with mesiobuccal cusp longer than distobuccal cusp, and no fifth cusp. Distolingual cusp smaller than on first or absent
Mesial contact: Middle third
Distal contact: Middle third
Distinguishing right from left: Mesiolingual cusp outline longer and larger but not as sharp as distolingual cusp
Root features: Trifurcated roots, with furcations, root trunks, and root concavities. Less divergent roots

Maxillary Right First Molar

CHARACTERISTICS:

Universal Number: #3
Eruption date: 6 years
General crown features: Occlusal table with marginal ridges, cusps with tips, inclined planes, ridges, grooves, fossae, and pits. Buccal cervical ridge
Specific crown features: Largest tooth in arch, largest crown in dentition. Four major cusps, with buccal cusps almost equal in height. Fifth minor cusp of Carabelli associated with mesiolingual cusp and prominent oblique ridge
Mesial contact: Junction of occulsal and middle thirds
Distal contact: Middle third
Distinguishing right from left: Mesiolingual cusp outline longer and larger but not as sharp as distolongual cusp
Root features: Trifurcated roots, with furcations, root trunks, and root concavities. Divergent roots. Furcations well removed from the CEJ

Maxillary Right Second Premolar

CHARACTERISTICS:

Universal Number: #4
Eruption date: 10-12 years
General crown features: Occlusal table with marginal ridges and cusps, with tips, ridges, inclined planes, grooves, fossae, pits. Buccal ridge
Specific crown features: Smaller than first, two cusps same length, short central groove, no mesial surface features like first, increased supplemental grooves
Mesial contact: Just cervical to the junction of occlusal and middle thirds
Distal contact: Just cervical to the junction of occlusal and middle thirds
Distinguishing right from left: Lingual cusp to offset to the mesial
General root features: Proximal root concavitites
Specific root features: Single-rooted. Elliptical on cross section

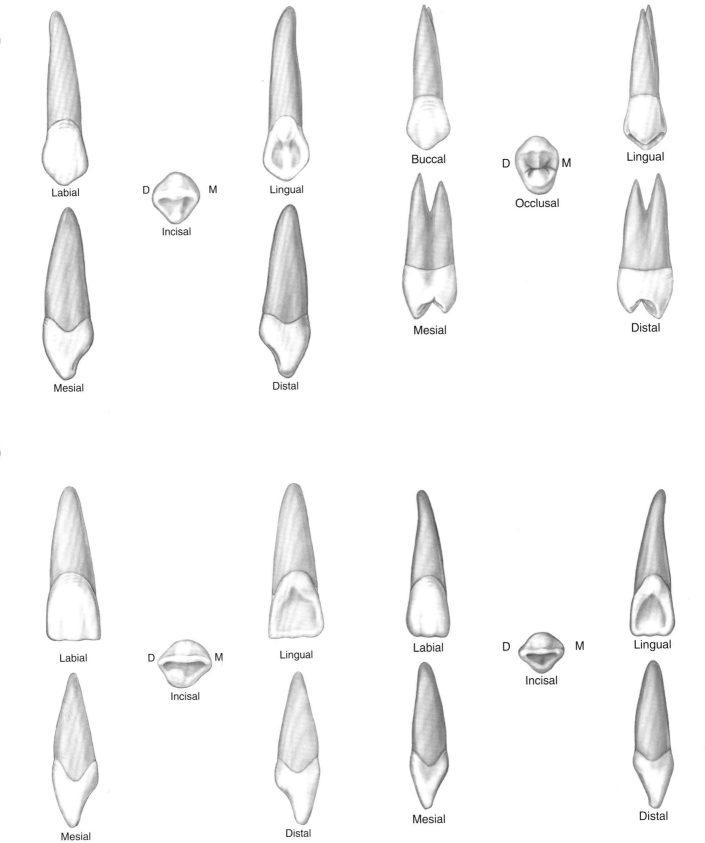

Labial

D ⊙ M
Incisal

Lingual

Mesial

Distal

Buccal

D ⊙ M
Occlusal

Lingual

Mesial

Distal

Labial

D ⊙ M
Incisal

Lingual

Mesial

Distal

Labial

D ⊙ M
Incisal

Lingual

Mesial

Distal

Maxillary Right First Premolar

CHARACTERISTICS:

Universal Number: #5
Eruption date: 10-11 years
General crown features: Occlusal table with marginal ridges and cusps, with tips, ridges, inclined planes, grooves, fossae, pits. Buccal ridge
Specific crown features: Larger than second, with buccal cusp longer of two, long central groove
Mesial contact: Just cervical to the junction of occlusal and middle thirds
Distal contact: Just cervical to the junction of occlusal and middle thirds
Distinguishing right from left: Longer mesial cusp slope, mesial features: marginal groove, developmental depression, deeper CEJ curvature
General root features: Proximal root concavities
Specific root features: Bifucated with root trunk. Elliptical on cross section

Maxillary Right Canine

CHARACTERISTICS:

Universal Number: #6
Eruption date: 11-12 years
General crown features: Single cusp, with tip and slopes, labial ridge, marginal ridges and lingual ridge, cingulum, and lingual fossae. Longest tooth in each arch or dentition
Specific crown features: Prominent lingual anatomy, sharp cusp tip
Height of contour: Labial: cervical third. Lingual: middle third
Mesial contact: Junction of incisal third and middle thirds
Distal contact: Middle third
Distinguishing right from left: Shorter mesial cusp slope, more cervical contact on distal, more pronounced mesial CEJ curvature. Shorter distal outline on labial view with depression between the distal contact and CEJ
General root features: Long, thick single root; ovoid on cross section; proximal root concavities
Specific root features: Blunt root apex

Maxillary Right Lateral Incisor

CHARACTERISTICS:

Universal Number: #7
Eruption date: 8-9 years
General crown features: Incisal edge and incisal angles
Specific crown features: Greatest crown variation, like a smaller maxillary central, prominent lingual surface. Centered cingulum, pronounced marginal ridges
Height of contour: Cervical third
Mesial contact: Incisal third
Distal contact: Middle third or junction with incisal third
Distinguishing right from left: Sharper MI angle, rounder DI angle, more pronounced mesial CEJ curvature
General root features: Single-rooted
Specific root features: Overall conical shape. No proximal root concavities. Root curves distally, with sharp apex. Oval in cross section. Same or longer than central but thinner

Maxillary Right Central Incisor

CHARACTERISTICS:

Universal Number: #8
Eruption date: 7-8 years
General crown features: Incisal edge and incisal angles
Specific crown features: Widest crown MD, greatest CEJ curve, and height of contour. Distal offset cingulum, shallow lingual fossa, marginal ridges
Height of contour: Cervical third
Mesial contact: Incisal third
Distal contact: Junction of incisal and middle thirds
Distinguishing right from left: Sharper MI angle, rounder DI angle, more pronounced mesial CEJ curvature
General root features: Single-rooted
Specific root features: Overall conical shape. No proximal root concavities. Rounded apex. Triangular in cross section

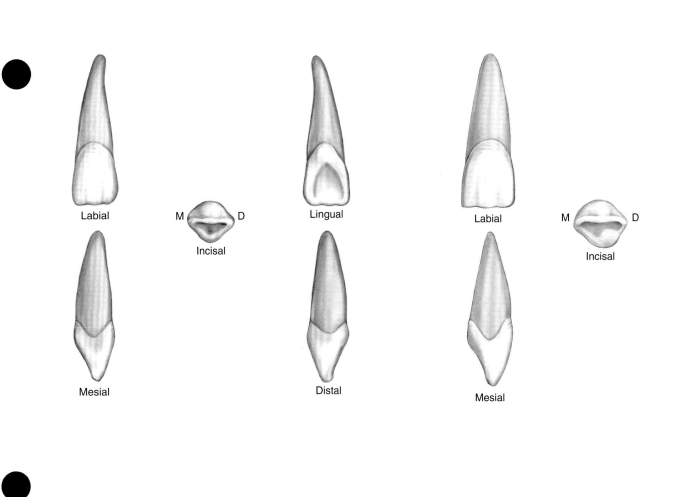

Labial   M ◯ D   Lingual

Incisal

Mesial   Distal

Labial   M ◯ D   Lingual

Incisal

Mesial   Distal

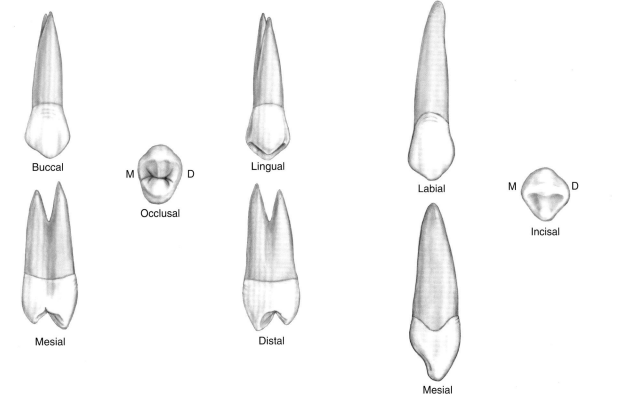

Buccal   M ◯ D   Lingual

Occlusal

Mesial   Distal

Labial   M ◯ D   Lingual

Incisal

Mesial   Distal

Maxillary Left Central Incisor

CHARACTERISTICS:

Universal Number: #9
Eruption date: 7-8 years
General crown features: Incisal edge and incisal angles
Specific crown features: Widest crown MD, greatest CEJ curve, and height of contour. Distal offset cingulum, shallow lingual fossa, marginal ridges
Height of contour: Cervical third
Mesial contact: Incisal third
Distal contact: Junction of incisal and middle thirds
Distinguishing right from left: Sharper MI angle, rounder DI angle, more pronounced mesial CEJ curvature
General root features: Single-rooted
Specific root features: Overall conical shape. No proximal root concavities. Rounded apex. Triangular in cross section

Maxillary Left Lateral Incisor

CHARACTERISTICS:

Universal Number: #10
Eruption date: 8-9 years
General crown features: Incisal edge and incisal angles
Specific crown features: Greatest crown variation, like a smaller maxillary central, prominent lingual surface. Centered cingulum, pronounced marginal ridges
Height of contour: Cervical third
Mesial contact: Incisal third
Distal contact: Middle third or junction with incisal third
Distinguishing right from left: Sharper MI angle, rounder DI angle, more pronounced mesial CEJ curvature
General root features: Single-rooted
Specific root features: Overall conical shape. No proximal root concavities. Root curves distally, with sharp apex. Oval in cross section. Same or longer than central but thinner

Maxillary Left Canine

CHARACTERISTICS:

Universal Number: #11
Eruption date: 11-12 years
General crown features: Single cusp, with tip and slopes, labial ridge, marginal ridges and lingual ridge, cingulum, and lingual fossae. Longest tooth in each arch or dentition
Specific crown features: Prominent lingual anatomy, sharp cusp tip
Height of contour: Labial: cervical third. Lingual: middle third
Mesial contact: Junction of incisal third and middle thirds
Distal contact: Middle third
Distinguishing right from left: Shorter mesial cusp slope, more cervical contact on distal, more pronounced mesial CEJ curvature. Shorter distal outline on labial view with depression between the distal contact and CEJ
General root features: Long, thick single root; ovoid on cross section; proximal root concavities
Specific root features: Blunt root apex

Maxillary Left First Premolar

CHARACTERISTICS:

Universal Number: #12
Eruption date: 10-11 years
General crown features: Occlusal table with marginal ridges and cusps, with tips, ridges, inclined planes, grooves, fossae, pits. Buccal ridge
Specific crown features: Larger than second, with buccal cusp longer of two, long central groove
Mesial contact: Just cervical to the junction of occlusal and middle thirds
Distal contact: Just cervical to the junction of occlusal and middle thirds
Distinguishing right from left: Longer mesial cusp slope, mesial features: marginal groove, developmental depression, deeper CEJ curvature
General root features: Proximal root concavities
Specific root features: Bifucated with root trunk. Elliptical on cross section

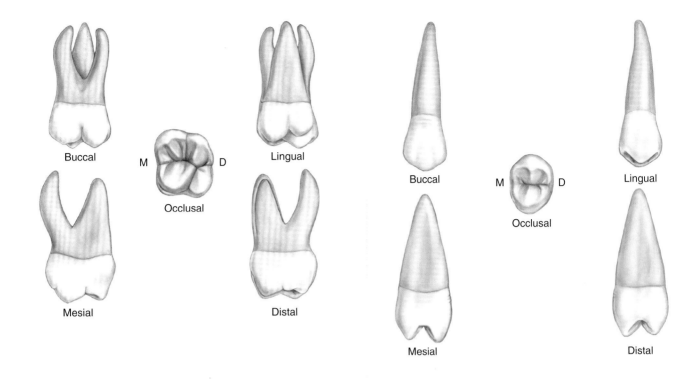

Buccal

M   D

Occlusal

Lingual

Mesial

Distal

Buccal

M   D

Occlusal

Lingual

Mesial

Distal

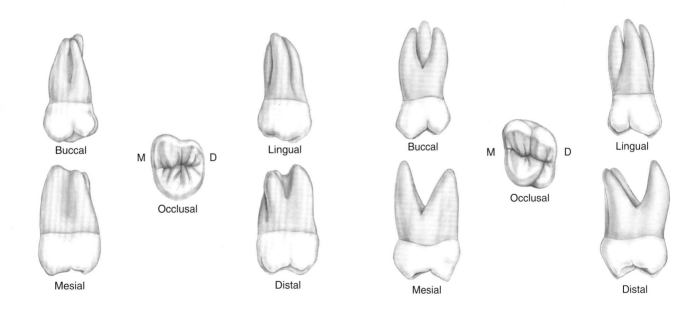

Buccal

M   D

Occlusal

Lingual

Mesial

Distal

Buccal

M   D

Occlusal

Lingual

Mesial

Distal

Maxillary Left Second Premolar

CHARACTERISTICS:

Universal Number: #13
Eruption date: 10-12 years
General crown features: Occlusal table with marginal ridges and cusps, with tips, ridges, inclined planes, grooves, fossae, pits. Buccal ridge
Specific crown features: Smaller than first, two cusps same length, short central groove, no mesial surface features like first, increased supplemental grooves
Mesial contact: Just cervical to the junction of occlusal and middle thirds
Distal contact: Just cervical to the junction of occlusal and middle thirds
Distinguishing right from left: Lingual cusp to offset to the mesial
General root features: Proximal root concavitites
Specific root features: Single-rooted. Elliptical on cross section

Maxillary Left First Molar

CHARACTERISTICS:

Universal Number: #14
Eruption date: 6 years
General crown features: Occlusal table with marginal ridges, cusps with tips, inclined planes, ridges, grooves, fossae, and pits. Buccal cervical ridge
Specific crown features: Largest tooth in arch, largest crown in dentition. Four major cusps, with buccal cusps almost equal in height. Fifth minor cusp of Carabelli associated with mesiolingual cusp and prominent oblique ridge
Mesial contact: Junction of occulsal and middle thirds
Distal contact: Middle third
Distinguishing right from left: Mesiolingual cusp outline longer and larger but not as sharp as distolongual cusp
Root features: Trifurcated roots, with furcations, root trunks, and root concavities. Divergent roots. Furcations well removed from the CEJ

Maxillary Left Second Molar (Rhombodial Crown Outline)

CHARACTERISTICS:

Universal Number: #15
Eruption date: 12-13 years
General crown features: Occlusal table with marginal ridges, cusps with tips, inclined planes, ridges, grooves, fossae, and pits. Buccal cervical ridge
Specific crown features: Smaller crown than first, heart-shaped or rhomboidal crown outline, thus three or four cusps. Oblique ridge less prominent, with mesiobuccal cusp longer than distobuccal cusp, and no fifth cusp. Distolingual cusp smaller than on first or absent
Mesial contact: Middle third
Distal contact: Middle third
Distinguishing right from left: Mesiolingual cusp outline longer and larger but not as sharp as distolingual cusp
Root features: Trifurcated roots, with furcations, root trunks, and root concavities. Less divergent roots

Maxillary Left Third Molar (Heart-shaped Occlusal Outline)

CHARACTERISTICS:

Universal Number: #16
Eruption date: 17-21 years
General crown features: Occlusal table with marginal ridges, cusps with tips, inclined planes, ridges, grooves, fossae, and pits. Buccal cervical ridge
Specific crown features: Smaller crown than second, variable in form, heart-shaped or rhomboidal crown outline, thus three or four cusps
Mesial contact: Middle third
Distal contact: None
Distinguishing right from left: Distobuccal cusp shorter than mesiobuccal cusp and roots curved distally
Root features: Usually fused roots, curving distally

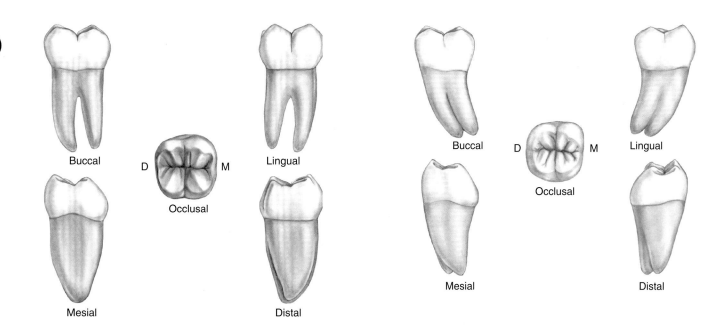

Buccal   D M   Lingual
Occlusal

Mesial   Distal

Buccal   D M   Lingual
Occlusal

Mesial   Distal

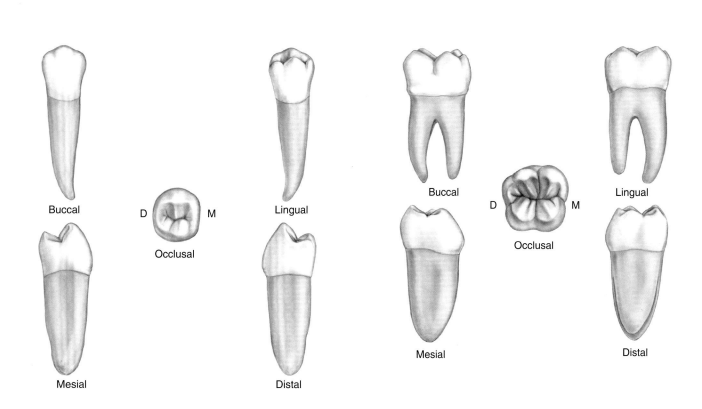

Buccal   D M   Lingual
Occlusal

Mesial   Distal

Buccal   D M   Lingual
Occlusal

Mesial   Distal

Mandibular Left Third Molar

CHARACTERISTICS:

Universal Number: #17
Eruption Date: 17-21 years
General crown features: Occlusal table with marginal ridges, cusps with tips, inclined planes, ridges, grooves, fossae, and pits
Specific crown features: Smaller crown than second
Mesial contact: Middle third
Distal contact: None
Distinguishing right from left: Wider buccolingually on mesial than on distal
General root features: Fused root, irregularly curved, with sharp apices

Mandibular Left Second Molar

CHARACTERISTICS:

Universal Number: #18
Eruption date: 11-13 years
General crown features: Occlusal table with marginal ridges, cusps with tips, inclined planes, ridges, grooves, fossae, and pits
Specific crown features: Smaller crown than first. Four cusps with cross-shaped groove pattern
Mesial contact: Middle third
Distal contact: Middle third
Distinguishing right from left: Difference in height of contour for buccal and lingual from each proximal surface, and wider on the mesial than distal
General root features: Bifurcated roots, with root trunks, furcation, and root concavities
Specific root features: Less divergent roots, with furcations closer to CEJ

Mandibular Left First Molar

CHARACTERISTICS:

Universal Number: #19
Eruption date: 6-7 years
General crown features: Occlusal table with marginal ridges, cusps with tips, inclined planes, ridges, grooves, fossae, and pits
Specific crown features: First permanent tooth to erupt, with widest crown mesiodistally of dentition. Five cusps, with Y groove pattern, and with buccal groove possibly ending in buccal pit
Mesial contact: Junction of occlusal and middle thirds
Distal contact: Junction of occlusal and middle thirds
Distinguishing right from left: Distal cusp is smallest and has a sharp cusp
General root features: Bifurcated roots, with root trunks, furcation, and root concavities
Specific root features: Divergent roots, with furcations well removed from the CEJ

Mandibular Left Second Premolar (Three Cusp Type)

CHARACTERISTICS:

Universal Number: #20
Eruption date: 11-12 years
General crown features: Occlusal table with marginal ridges and cusps, with tips, ridges, inclined planes, grooves, fossae, pits. Buccal ridge
Specific crown features: Larger than first, usually three cusps: Y groove pattern or two cusps: H or U groove pattern, increased supplemental grooves
Mesial contact: Just cervical to the junction of occlusal and middle thirds
Distal contact: Just cervical to the junction of occlusal and middle thirds
Distinguishing right from left: Distal marginal ridge more cervically located, thus more occlusal surface visible from distal view
General root features: Proximal root concavities
Specific root features: Single-rooted. Ovoid or elliptical on cross section

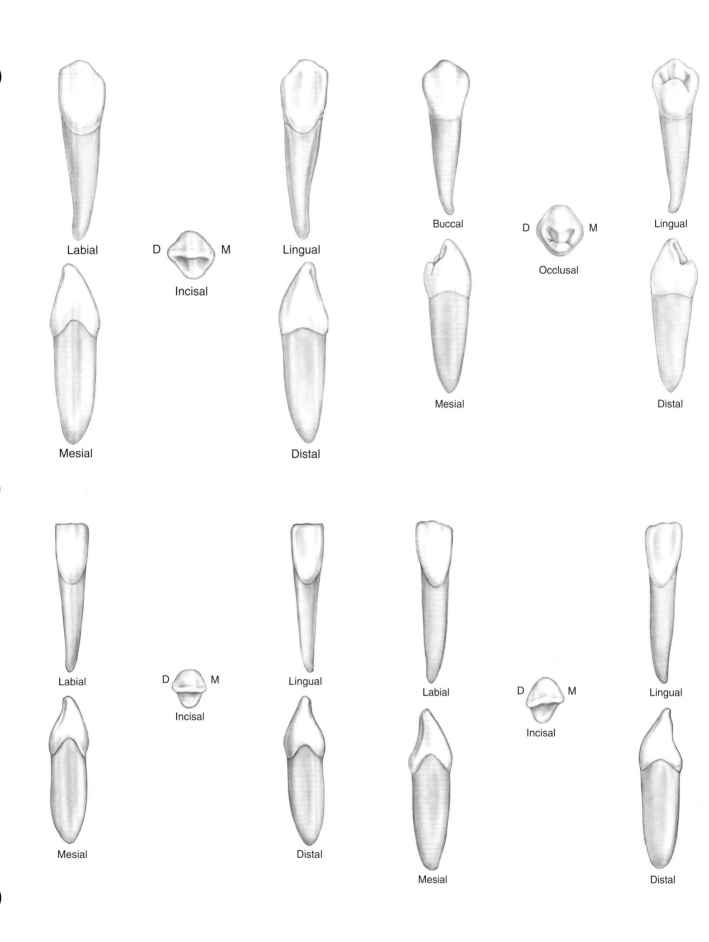

Labial

D   M
Incisal

Lingual

Mesial

Distal

Buccal

D   M
Occlusal

Lingual

Mesial

Distal

Labial

D   M
Incisal

Lingual

Mesial

Distal

Labial

D   M
Incisal

Lingual

Mesial

Distal

Mandibular Left First Premolar

CHARACTERISTICS:

Universal Number: #21
Eruption date: 10-12 years
General crown features: Occlusal table with marginal ridges and cusps, with tips, ridges, inclined planes, grooves, fossae, pits. Buccal ridge
Specific crown features: Smaller than second, smaller lingual cusp of two, mesial surfacefeatures
Mesial contact: Just cervical to the junction of occlusal and middle thirds
Distal contact: Just cervical to the junction of occlusal and middle thirds
Distinguishing right from left: Shorter mesial cusp slope, mesiolingual groove, deeper mesial CEJ curvature
General root features: Proximal root concavities
Specific root features: Single-rooted. Ovoid or elliptical on cross section

Mandibular Left Canine

CHARACTERISTICS:

Universal Number: #22
Eruption date: 9-10 years
General crown features: Single cusp, with tip and slopes, labial ridge, marginal ridges and lingual ridge, cingulum, and lingual fossae. Longest tooth in each arch or dentition
Specific crown features: Smoother lingual anatomy, less sharp cusp tip
Height of contour: Labial: cervical third. Lingual: middle third
Mesial contact: Incisal third
Distal contact: Junction of incisal and middle thirds
Distinguishing right from left: Shorter mesial cusp slope, more cervical contact on distal, more pronounced mesial CEJ curvature. Shorter and rounder distal outline on labial view, with a shorter mesial slope than distal
General root features: Long, thick single root; ovoid on cross section; proximal root concavities
Specific root features: Developmental depressions on mesial and distal give tooth double-rooted appearance. Pointed apex

Mandibular Left Lateral Incisor

CHARACTERISTICS:

Universal Number: #23
Eruption date: 7-8 years
General crown features: Incisal edge and incisal angles
Specific crown features: Like a larger mandibular central, not bilaterally symmetrical. Appears twisted distally. Small, distally placed cingulum; lingual fossa and moderate mesial marginal ridge longer than distal
Height of contour: Cervical third
Mesial contact: Incisal third
Distal contact: Incisal third
Distinguishing right from left: Sharper MI angle, rounder DI angle, more pronounced mesial CEJ curvature
General root features: Single-rooted
Specific root features: Bow shaped on cross section. Root is longer than the crown. Proximal root concavities give double-rooted appearance

Mandibular Left Central Incisor

CHARACTERISTICS:

Universal Number: #24
Eruption date: 6-7 years
General crown features: Incisal edge and incisal angles
Specific crown features: Smallest and simplest tooth, bilaterally symmetrical. Small centered cingulum, subtle lingual fossa, and equal subtle marginal ridges
Height of contour: Cervical third
Mesial contact: Incisal third
Distal contact: Incisal third
Distinguishing right from left: Sharper MI angle, rounder DI angle, more pronounced mesial CEJ curvature
General root features: Single-rooted
Specific root features: Bow shaped on cross section. Root is longer than the crown. Proximal root concavities give double-rooted appearance

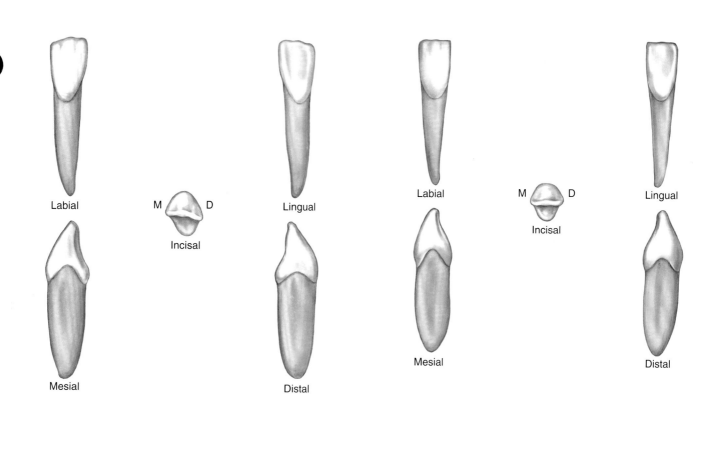

Labial   M Incisal D   Lingual

Mesial   Distal

Labial   M Incisal D   Lingual

Mesial   Distal

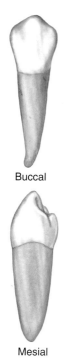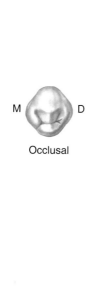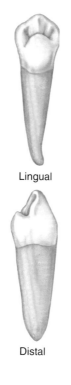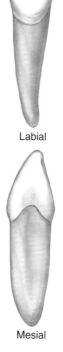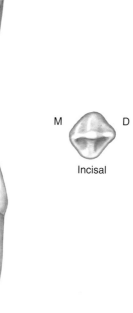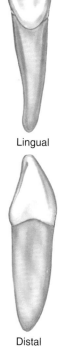

Buccal   M Occlusal D   Lingual

Mesial   Distal

Labial   M Incisal D   Lingual

Mesial   Distal

Mandibular Right Central Incisor

CHARACTERISTICS:

Universal Number: #25
Eruption date: 6-7 years
General crown features: Incisal edge and incisal angles
Specific crown features: Smallest and simplest tooth, bilaterally symmetrical. Small centered cingulum, subtle lingual fossa, and equal subtle marginal ridges
Height of contour: Cervical third
Mesial contact: Incisal third
Distal contact: Incisal third
Distinguishing right from left: Sharper MI angle, rounder DI angle, more pronounced mesial CEJ curvature
General root features: Single-rooted
Specific root features: Bow shaped on cross section. Root is longer than the crown. Proximal root concavities give double-rooted appearance

Mandibular Right Lateral Incisor

CHARACTERISTICS:

Universal Number: #26
Eruption date: 7-8 years
General crown features: Incisal edge and incisal angles
Specific crown features: Like a larger mandibular central, not bilaterally symmetrical. Appears twisted distally. Small, distally placed cingulum; lingual fossa and moderate mesial marginal ridge longer than distal
Height of contour: Cervical third
Mesial contact: Incisal third
Distal contact: Incisal third
Distinguishing right from left: Sharper MI angle, rounder DI angle, more pronounced mesial CEJ curvature
General root features: Single-rooted
Specific root features: Bow shaped on cross section. Root is longer than the crown. Proximal root concavities give double-rooted appearance

Mandibular Right Canine

CHARACTERISTICS:

Universal Number: #27
Eruption date: 9-10 years
General crown features: Single cusp, with tip and slopes, labial ridge, marginal ridges and lingual ridge, cingulum, and lingual fossae. Longest tooth in each arch or dentition
Specific crown features: Smoother lingual anatomy, less sharp cusp tip
Height of contour: Labial: cervical third. Lingual: middle third
Mesial contact: Incisal third
Distal contact: Junction of incisal and middle thirds
Distinguishing right from left: Shorter mesial cusp slope, more cervical contact on distal, more pronounced mesial CEJ curvature. Shorter and rounder distal outline on labial view, with a shorter mesial slope than distal
General root features: Long, thick single root; ovoid on cross section; proximal root concavities
Specific root features: Developmental depressions on mesial and distal give tooth double-rooted appearance. Pointed apex

Mandibular Right First Premolar

CHARACTERISTICS:

Universal Number: #28
Eruption date: 10-12 years
General crown features: Occlusal table with marginal ridges and cusps, with tips, ridges, inclined planes, grooves, fossae, pits. Buccal ridge.
Specific crown features: Smaller than second, smaller lingual cusp of two, mesial surface features
Mesial contact: Just cervical to the junction of occlusal and middle thirds
Distal contact: Just cervical to the junction of occlusal and middle thirds
Distinguishing right from left: Shorter mesial cusp slope, mesiolingual groove, deeper mesial CEJ curvature
General root features: Proximal root concavities
Specific root features: Single-rooted. Ovoid or elliptical on cross section

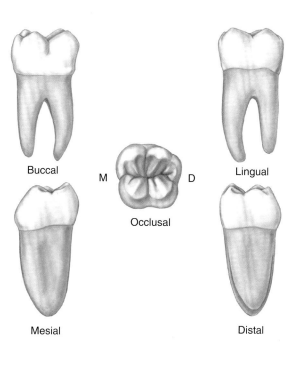

Buccal

M   D

Occlusal

Lingual

Mesial

Distal

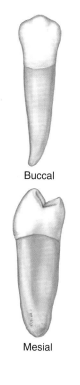

Buccal

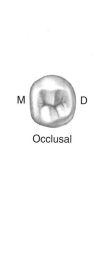

M   D

Occlusal

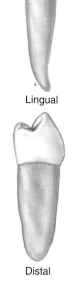

Lingual

Mesial

Distal

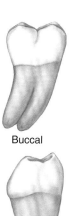

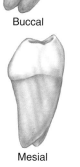

Buccal

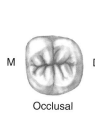

M   D

Occlusal

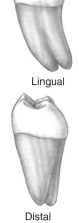

Lingual

Mesial

Distal

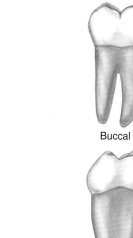

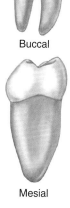

Buccal

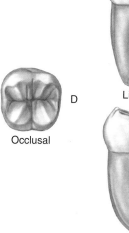

M   D

Occlusal

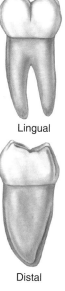

Lingual

Mesial

Distal

Mandibular Right Second Premolar (Three Cusp Type)

CHARACTERISTICS:

Universal Number: #29
Eruption date: 11-12 years
General crown features: Occlusal table with marginal ridges and cusps, with tips, ridges, inclined planes, grooves, fossae, pits. Buccal ridge
Specific crown features: Larger than first, usually three cusps: Y groove pattern or two cusps: H or U groove pattern, increased supplemental grooves
Mesial contact: Just cervical to the junction of occlusal and middle thirds
Distal contact: Just cervical to the junction of occlusal and middle thirds
Distinguishing right from left: Distal marginal ridge more cervically located, thus more occlusal surface visible from distal view
General root features: Proximal root concavities
Specific root features: Single-rooted. Ovoid or elliptical on cross section

Mandibular Right First Molar

CHARACTERISTICS:

Universal Number: #30
Eruption date: 6-7 years
General crown features: Occlusal table with marginal ridges, cusps with tips, inclined planes, ridges, grooves, fossae, and pits
Specific crown features: First permanent tooth to erupt, with widest crown mesiodistally of dentition. Five cusps, with Y groove pattern, and with buccal groove possibly ending in buccal pit
Mesial contact: Junction of occlusal and middle thirds
Distal contact: Junction of occlusal and middle thirds
Distinguishing right from left: Distal cusp is smallest and has a sharp cusp
General root features: Bifurcated roots, with root trunks, furcation, and root concavities
Specific root features: Divergent roots, with furcations well removed from the CEJ

Mandibular Right Second Molar

CHARACTERISTICS:

Universal Number: #31
Eruption date: 11-13 years
General crown features: Occlusal table with marginal ridges, cusps with tips, inclined planes, ridges, grooves, fossae, and pits
Specific crown features: Smaller crown than first. Four cusps with cross-shaped groove pattern
Mesial contact: Middle third
Distal contact: Middle third
Distinguishing right from left: Difference in height of contour for buccal and lingual from each proximal surface, and wider on the mesial than distal
General root features: Bifurcated roots, with root trunks, furcation, and root concavities
Specific root features: Less divergent roots, with furcations closer to CEJ

Mandibular Right Third Molar

CHARACTERISTICS:

Universal Number: #32
Eruption date: 17-21 years
General crown features: Occlusal table with marginal ridges, cusps with tips, inclined planes, ridges, grooves, fossae, and pits
Specific crown features: Smaller crown than second
Mesial contact: Middle third
Distal contact: None
Distinguishing right from left: Wider buccolingually on mesial than on distal
General root features: Fused root, irregularly curved, with sharp apices